21 SECRET REMEDIES FOR COLDS AND FLU

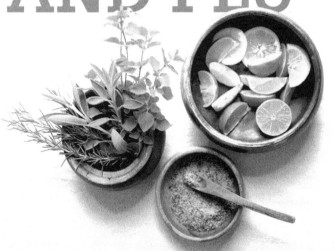

Most CHARISMA HOUSE BOOK GROUP products are available at special quantity discounts for bulk purchase for sales promotions, premiums, fund-raising, and educational needs. For details, write Charisma House Book Group, 600 Rinehart Road, Lake Mary, Florida 32746, or telephone (407) 333-0600.

21 SECRET REMEDIES FOR COLDS AND FLU edited by Siloam
Published by Siloam
Charisma Media/Charisma House Book Group
600 Rinehart Road
Lake Mary, Florida 32746
www.charismahouse.com

Cover design by Justin Evans

For more information on books published by Siloam, visit www .charismahouse.com.

Library of Congress Cataloging-in-Publication Data:
An application to register this book for cataloging has been submitted to the Library of Congress.
International Standard Book Number: 978-1-62998-010-2
E-book ISBN: 978-1-62998-011-9

This book contains the opinions and ideas of its authors. It is solely for informational and educational purposes and should not be regarded as a substitute for professional medical treatment. The nature of your body's health condition is complex and unique. Therefore, you should consult a health professional before you begin any new exercise, nutrition, or supplementation program or if you have questions about your health. Neither the authors nor the publisher shall be liable or responsible for any loss or damage allegedly arising from any information or suggestion in this book.

The statements in this book about consumable products or food have not been evaluated by the Food and Drug Administration. The recipes in this book are to be followed exactly as written. The publisher is not responsible for your specific health or allergy needs that may require medical supervision. The publisher is not responsible for any adverse reactions to the consumption of food or products that have been suggested in this book.

First edition

15 16 17 18 19 — 987654321
Printed in the United States of America

CONTENTS

INTRODUCTION

REGARDLESS OF WHERE you live, after the recent nasty winters that have affected even those living in the more southerly regions of the United States, the onset of winter often produces the dreaded thought of colds, flu, and other dangerous viruses floating through the air. They can be deadly: flu is linked to about twenty thousand deaths in the United States annually, and about one hundred thirty thousand people go to a hospital each year with the flu. So it's no wonder that when people think about the possibilities of colds and flu, they often say, "Yeech!"

As much as we dislike these imbalances and their effects, though, natural medicine practitioners see a cold as your body's attempt to cleanse itself of toxins, wastes, bacteria, and mucus that have built up to the point of overwhelming the immune system. The same is true with influenza (or flu), which is an acute viral infection of the upper respiratory tract or digestive tract caused by a rhinovirus. The flu can begin with symptoms that resemble the common cold, but the infection is generally more severe, highly contagious, and longer lasting. Besides lingering fatigue and weakness, influenza can make a person more susceptible to pneumonia, sinus problems, bronchitis, and ear infections. People older than sixty can be seriously affected by the flu, which is the fifth-leading cause of death in the elderly.

However, fighting colds and flu starts long before the thermometer plunges. There are many commonsense, natural methods you can take to build your body's immunity. Prevention starts with eating healthy foods such as mushrooms, vegetables, oats, and peppers, and avoiding bad ones, particularly sugar. Vitamins, minerals, and supplements help supply your body with substances often missing from the modern diet. Good hygiene habits, such as washing your hands regularly and caring for your skin and teeth, will reduce your chances of getting sick. So will getting adequate sleep and rest, reducing stress levels, and incorporating outdoor activity into your lifestyle. Getting outside during good weather provides you with more sunshine-induced vitamin D and puts you in touch with the soil and other healthy aspects of nature. Lowering your weight, cholesterol levels, and blood pressure will also leave you less susceptible to viruses.

Exercise is another preventive measure that will lessen your chances of coming down with colds or flu during bad weather. So will a positive mental outlook. Staying in touch with friends and loved ones, and taking time to laugh (and pray) each day will help you avoid the loneliness and depression that afflict millions in American society. A body weakened by "the blues" is more susceptible to viruses of all kinds, which is why you need to get regular checkups, so you can confide in your doctor about any personal problems that may be affecting your overall health.

Even if all these measures fail and you wind up getting sick, avoid reaching for the nearest over-the-counter medication. There are many natural remedies that can help cure what ails you, without adverse side effects. We have sought to compile a quick reference guide to help you the next time you find yourself concerned about cold and flu season. Hopefully, armed with good information, you will be able to avoid the "yeechs" that sideline too many people.

Chapter 1

KNOW YOUR ENVIRONMENT

E VER SINCE THE Industrial Revolution we have poured dangerous chemicals and pollutants into our streams, soil, and air. As a result, through both food and environment, you are exposed daily to pesticides, food additives, solvents, and other chemicals and hazardous substances.

For example, at this moment you probably have some amount of lead in your body, usually stored in your bones.[1] Most people have small amounts of DDT (or its metabolite DDE, which is what it changes into during metabolism) in their fatty tissues. Lead, one of the most commonly used metals (other than iron), is used for manufacturing batteries, chemicals, and other metal products. Lead has contaminated our entire planet, landing in some of the most remote areas on the planet.

Such toxic exposure can put us at hazard of fatal diseases such as cancer and, more commonly, sicknesses such as colds and flu. While these are seemingly inconsequential, we mentioned in the introduction that the flu is the fifth-leading cause of death in people over age sixty. Awareness of toxicity in your environment is the first step to reducing the substances and influences that can land you in a sickbed.

INGESTING TOXINS

Today going to the doctor and getting antibiotics at the first sign of the sniffles is about as common as eating a peanut butter sandwich. Don't be too quick to do this. If you have had repeated bouts of antibiotics, or even a single bout of super antibiotics, then you could be at risk for developing an overgrowth of yeast and dangerous intestinal bacteria.

To explain, your intestines are filled with good bacteria called *lactobacillus acidophilus* and *bifidus* that prevent the overgrowth of bad bacteria (called *pathogenic bacteria* or *microbes*) in your intestinal tract. When you take antibiotics, these medications can kill many of your body's beneficial bacteria. Your good bacteria function like a firewall to

1

keep pathogenic bacteria and yeast in check. So when antibiotics throw off the balance, the bad or pathogenic bacteria may grow like a wildfire—out of control with nothing to slow it down or stop it. Now your body is in trouble, for bad bacteria may produce endotoxins. These dangerous substances may be as toxic as almost any chemical, pesticide, or solvent that enters your body from outside.

ADDRESSING YOUR ENVIRONMENT

Numerous toxic substances populate the modern world. Reducing exposure to them will improve your health, boost your mental outlook, and leave you feeling cleaner—inside and out. This involves everything from hazards in the outside environment to pesticides lying around the average home. You can address these through a variety of precautions and proactive steps.

First, let's review a few of the environmental contaminants that can weaken your immune system and adversely affect your health.

Air pollution

While particularly bad in metropolitan areas, poor air quality affects rural communities too. Even small-town residents know the familiar smell of gasoline fumes. Avoid them—and the smog they help produce. Travelers who wait for a taxi or bus at the airport should do so inside, away from traffic fumes. At a bus station, don't stand behind the buses. Motorists should never sit in heavy traffic with the window open. In addition, if you are following a motorist whose car emits a cloud of nauseating fumes, take another route if possible. Those dangerous emissions are high in carbon monoxide, hydrocarbons, and other chemical pollutants. If you can't take an alternate route, roll up your windows and drive a safe distance away from the vehicle while recycling the air in your car.

A word to joggers and bicyclists: never jog, run, or ride alongside a busy highway where your lungs can absorb high amounts of carbon monoxide, hydrocarbons, and other toxins.

Oil spills

If you smell gas or see smoke from oil burns, stay indoors. Also, set your air conditioner to recycle the indoor air so the outdoor air doesn't filter into the house. Avoid physical exertion that puts extra demands on your lungs and heart.

Follow local and state public health guidelines for consumption of seafood and water affected by petroleum spills. Stay up-to-date on local and state public health guidelines on water activities, such as swimming, boating, and fishing.

Extended contact with oil dispersants can cause rashes, dry skin, and eye irritations. If you experience prolonged exposure to oil dispersants, see your doctor immediately.[2]

Nuclear radiation

Nuclear power plants and other sources of radiation are part of twenty-first-century life. When exposed to nuclear radiation, pay attention to three principles: time, distance, and shielding.[3]

The amount of exposure increases and decreases according to time spent near the source. If radioactive material gets inside your body, you aren't able to move away from it.

Concerning distance, the farther away from the source, the less the exposure. Alpha and beta particles aren't strong enough to travel far, but gamma rays can travel long distances and create the need to be especially careful of exposure distance.

As a general rule, doubling your distance from the radioactive source will reduce its exposure power by a factor of four. In general the greater the shield you have from a radioactive source, the less exposure you have to it. The shield absorbs the radiation between you and the source, and the amount of shielding required depends on the amount of energy given off by the rays. A thin material, such as paper, is strong enough to shield against alpha particles. Heavy clothing is sufficient for beta particles. But a much heavier, dense shield, such as lead, is necessary for protection against powerful gamma rays.

Other Solutions

Sick building syndrome

You can minimize "sick building syndrome" (more about this in chapter 18) in your home by choosing less toxic carpets or installing hardwood floors or tile floors. Use less toxic paints. Never buy or use furniture made of pressed wood or particleboard. Instead, choose hardwood or metal furniture. Select drapes made of cotton instead of fabrics treated with formaldehyde.

Also, consider the medicinal and mental value of plants. Not only do they create an attractive environment, but plants also have a practical use: they take in carbon dioxide and other dangerous gases and give off clean, pure oxygen. If you suspect the office building where you work is sick, surround your work space with plants. Spider plants, philodendrons, Boston ferns, and English ivy are all easy-to-grow, hardy indoor plants. Best yet, they tend to be excellent natural air purifiers.

Bacteria, mold, and yeast

Minimize your exposure to mold spores and dust mites by keeping the heating and air-conditioning ducts in your home clean. Set up a schedule for periodic cleaning and stick with it.

In addition, lower the relative humidity in your home to less than 50 percent. This will discourage the growth of mold and dust mites. Take special note of the rooms that tend to be most damp, such as the bathroom and laundry room.

If you live in a very humid climate, consider purchasing a dehumidifier for your home. Use an air purifier, such as a hepa filter or ionizer air filter, to remove chemicals and toxins in the air. Open the windows and doors in your home during the day to get fresh air. Open the windows or doors in your office as well to get fresh air and to dilute some of the toxic air. Turn the ceiling fan on with a window open; there is even a better exchange for outside air. Be sure to dust the top of the fan periodically.

Pesticide pollution

One of the most important ways you can reduce your exposure to pesticides is to stop having your home sprayed. Try more natural methods of bug control, such as sprinkling cupboards and closets with boric acid.

In addition, avoid the use of air fresheners or air deodorizers. Try more natural air fresheners, such as a pot of fragrant flowers on your dining room table. Better yet, open your windows on cool mornings and evenings to air out your home. If you have a window that catches a regular breeze, try planting fragrant flowers such as jasmine nearby. Aromatic plants can refresh your home with a lovely, natural scent while at the same time providing natural air purifiers and fresh oxygen.

While some may react negatively to this request, ask everyone to take their shoes off before coming inside from outdoors. This is a major way that pesticides enter your home. House dust can accumulate large amounts of pesticides that have been tracked in from outside. Daily vacuuming just tends to send them into the air, making the situation even worse. It is much simpler to cultivate the habit of asking everyone visiting your home to remove their shoes.

Chapter 2

KNOW THE TRUTH

I N THE UNITED States alone there are an estimated one billion colds every year, usually occurring between October and March. The average adult contracts two to four colds annually while the average child gets six to ten. Indeed, nothing is more miserable than getting a cold or flu. But did you know the reason we suffer so much is because we do all the wrong things when we get sick? Drinking coffee and sodas and eating ice cream and pudding can make your flu or cold worse—or prolong it. Don't count on a flu shot offering ironclad protection, either. Flu shots have not been as successful as hoped because viral strains constantly change and make one year's vaccine virtually obsolete the next.

However, when it comes to colds and flu, recognize that few topics are the source of so many myths. For example, many believe that colds are caused by cold weather, and that not dressing properly for weather conditions will lead to illness. Another mistaken belief is that a person must be ill or have a weakened immune system to be susceptible to colds. The truth is that colds are caused by viruses. In order to get sick from the viruses that cause colds, you must come into contact with them. They must attach to your cells and multiply within your cells to cause infection. Although not dressing properly for the weather conditions is not a good idea, there is no evidence you can contract a cold because of it.

Second, a person need not have a weakened immune system to be susceptible to cold viruses. In one study involving healthy adults, 95 percent became infected when cold viruses were administered through the nose.[1] Of those, a large percentage developed symptoms associated with the common cold. More than two hundred viruses are known to cause colds. Indeed, there are so many different types or strains of cold viruses it is difficult to develop a vaccine to provide protection from all of them.

Unlike what many think about the transmission of colds, the viruses that cause them are usually transmitted by direct contact with the hands.

6

The hands then touch the mouth, nose, or eyes, and the virus multiplies in the nose. The symptoms are probably the result of the body's immune response to the virus. This causes inflammation in the lining of the nose, resulting in sneezing and a blocked, runny nose. Fluid may drain from the nose to the throat, causing soreness, and from the back of the throat to the chest, causing coughing.

The Truth About Flu

Many people have similar misconceptions about the flu. One is the belief they can contract the flu from cold weather. Another is that you must be sick to be susceptible. There is also the belief that the symptoms of a cold can become so severe it can develop into the flu. The truth: the flu is also a respiratory infection caused by viruses. Just as with cold viruses, you must be exposed to the flu virus to become infected. It is not transmitted via cold weather, nor is it necessary to be sick to become infected. Unless a person is infected with both cold and flu viruses, it is unlikely that a cold will develop into the flu. It is more likely that the symptoms of a severe cold and the flu are so similar it is difficult for many to distinguish between the two.

There are three types of viruses that cause the flu: influenza types A, B, and C. Influenza type A is further classified into two groups based on their types of surface proteins that are recognized by our immune systems. Influenza types A and B viruses are the most common cause of disease. Influenza type C causes less severe respiratory infections and is usually not involved in epidemics. The type A influenza virus has also been found in animals, including birds, pigs, and whales.

The mode of transmission for flu viruses is respiratory droplets from sneezes and coughs. An infected person may sneeze or cough, and droplets carrying the virus may get on the mouth or nose of a person in close proximity. This gives the virus access to the cells of the respiratory tract, thus causing illness. Adults may be contagious before symptoms and are capable of spreading the germs for up to seven days after symptoms appear. Children may be contagious for several days before the onset of symptoms and may be contagious for ten days or more afterward. Persons with compromised immune systems may spread viruses for months.

Symptoms from the flu are usually far more severe and occur quickly after infection. In addition to the common cold symptoms, flu symptoms include high fever (above 102 degrees Fahrenheit), headaches, body aches, muscle aches, and tiredness. Sometimes people with the flu contract secondary infections, causing complications. Some examples are bacterial pneumonia, ear and sinus infections, and worsening of long-term chronic illnesses.

The Natural Way

When you come down with a cold or flu, fast by drinking plenty of water and fresh juices, and get lots of rest.

Jump-Start Juicing

For those who want to join the healthy trend of juicing as a cold and flu fighter, here is a list of ingredients that will help jump-start the habit. This will give you enough to juice for about a week (prepare daily).

  5–10 pounds organic carrots

  7 lemons or limes, or 3 or 4 of each

  7 cucumbers

  1 bunch celery

  2 bunches chard or collard greens

  1 bunch parsley

  1 big ginger root

  7 apples (green are lower in sugar)

This will help your system to expel toxic materials through the mucus it creates. Let your fever burn up your infection too. A fever mobilizes your immune system to fight infections. However, most physicians and parents turn off a fever with Tylenol and deplete levels of glutathione, a master antioxidant and detoxifier found in such supplements as folate and vitamins B_6 and B_{12}. Don't rush to the doctor and take a lot of medications to halt the symptoms. Some are important for detoxification. (However, if you have a fever over 103 degrees, you should be examined by a physician.)

As mentioned in chapter 1, when you are sick, don't instantly turn to antibiotics. Although they can provide powerful help when you are suffering from a bacterial infection, antibiotics' overuse can harm you. Plus, since colds and flu stem from viruses, antibiotics cannot kill them. In addition, when antibiotics are used too frequently, bacteria can develop immunity to the antibiotic. Today our nation is seeing increasing numbers of antibiotic-resistant strains of bacteria because of overprescribing them. This weakens the immune system and makes you more vulnerable to repeated illness.

Quick Tips: Fighting or Preventing Illness

If seeking to build your immune system or you are bothered by a cold or the flu, try these natural substances:

- Astragalus: This is a natural dietary supplement.
- Cayenne (capsicum): Hot chili peppers, or red pepper in its powdered form, are one of nature's remedies for these ailments. They also will fight infections and sore throats.
- Echinacea (coneflower): Boosts white blood cell production and immune system support.
- Goldenseal: Prevents colds, flu, and sore throats from developing.
- Stevia: This natural sweetener can also prevent colds and flu. Users of stevia-enhanced products report a lower incidence of these ailments.

- For juices that will help fight sickness, try blending carrots with: 1) beet and cucumber, 2) celery and radish, or 3) spinach.
- Homemade chicken soup
- Drink plenty of fluids, including water with lemon, green tea, and diluted fruit juices.

Try alternative remedies, such as taking plenty of vitamin C. Garlic, elderberry, and herbs, such as olive leaf extract and oregano, are a natural means to help your body's immune response. In addition, using an infrared sauna helps boost the immune system. You can overcome many infectious diseases by eliminating mucus-forming foods, such as dairy products, eggs, and processed grains. These grains include pancakes, cereals, doughnuts, white bread, crackers, pretzels, bagels, white rice, gravies, cakes, and pies. You should also shun margarine, butter, and other saturated, hydrogenated, and processed oils.

Recipe: Immune System Building

Vitamin C is an important nutrient for the immune system, your body's leading line of defense against infectious diseases. This recipe makes two servings.

1 green apple
1/2 cucumber, peeled if not organic
2-3 leaves kale or collard greens
1 handful parsley or watercress
1 cup elderberries or blueberries
1 lemon, peeled if not organic

Cut produce to fit your juicer's feed tube. Wrap parsley or watercress in the green leaves and push through the juicer slowly with half of the cucumber. Turn off the machine and pour in the berries, then place the plunger on top. Turn the machine on and push the berries through. Juice all remaining ingredients. Stir the juice and drink as soon as possible.

FIRST LINE OF DEFENSE

Let your body's immune system be your first defense. When it comes to colds, flu, and sinus infections, your skin and mucous membranes are powerful defenders. Viruses and bacteria cannot penetrate the skin unless entering through a cut or break. That's when an inflammatory response occurs, which sends your immune system into high gear to rid the body of the bacteria or virus. Cold and flu viruses enter the body through the mucous membranes, creating inflammation and swelling. Swollen, inflamed mucous membranes cause the mucous glands to secrete more mucus as they rid the body of the virus. But too much swelling can block off sinus openings so that they cannot drain. Stagnant mucus then becomes infected with bacteria, creating a sinus infection.

One of the keys to fighting these "space invaders" is appreciating the amazing nature of the immune system God built into your body to ward off viruses, bacteria, parasites, fungi, and much more. There are many other immune system components in this stunning arsenal of defense, such as interleukins and interferons. A healthy, intact immune system can take on even the most deadly assaults. Colds, flu, and sinus infections pose little challenge to a healthy, well-functioning immune system operating at peak efficiency.

Chapter 3

SLEEP AND REST

Most Americans live hectic, stressful lives. People who live under stressful conditions appear to be more susceptible to infections than people living under less stressful conditions. That is why getting proper rest is an important part of caring for your body. You cannot expect your body to work hard to defend you from colds, flu, and other infectious diseases if you do not take care of it. This means setting aside time to rest. The Word of God says people should not work continuously, but rather set aside specific time for this purpose. After all, a refreshed body is more equipped to work for you.

Chapter 2 mentioned that most colds and flu occur between October and March. It's interesting, then, that every winter many animals hibernate or rest for a season. Likewise, every night when you sleep, you rest your body and mind. Blessed rest is as much a law of the universe as gravity. It is also a powerful principle of healing. Think about it: When an animal is injured or sick, what does it do? It finds a resting place where it can lap up water and quit eating while it heals. This is a natural, instinctual wisdom that God placed within the animal kingdom.

But when many people come down with an illness, such as a bad cold or sinus infection, what do they do? Instead of resting and fasting by drinking only water or fresh-made juices, they consume ice cream, puddings, creamy soups, and other rich, high-caloric foods that do nothing to cleanse and detoxify the body. Many also prolong illnesses by taking Tylenol to suppress the fever so they can go back to work much sooner than their bodies are ready (often sickening coworkers in the process). They push themselves by taking antibiotics, decongestants, and antihistamines to dry up the mucus. This also impedes the natural process of detoxification. Instead of healing, the body may store even more toxic material.

Tapping in to Strength

Those who sleep better and know how to rest or meditate can tap in to creativity, new ideas, and a spiritual state much faster than those who try to get by with little rest. Basically a good night's sleep is like pushing "reset" on your computer when it goes haywire. Rest is an integral element of good health, which includes being free of disease, injury, and stress. Your overall health depends greatly on the decisions you make. God grants each person the option to choose. You can choose to get adequate rest, as well as eating right, exercising, and decreasing the stress in your life.

Practicing healthy behaviors contributes to your well-being and can greatly reduce the risk of infections and illness. However, Americans' record on the sleep meter isn't too good. Over the past five decades people's average nightly sleep declined from more than eight hours to less than seven. To show how this compounds health problems, during this same span of time the nation's obesity rate climbed 30 percent. Less sleep means lower levels of leptin, the hormone that tells you that you have eaten enough.

Here is where lifestyle choices, including exercise, will help you get more rest. For example, in addition to stretching in the morning and starting a regular jogging or walking program, stretching before going to bed at night will help to relax you and promote more restful sleep. You will be surprised at how great it makes you feel. As you continue, you will see that you can walk faster and for longer periods of time with positive results. Limiting your intake of caffeine, whether that is through coffee, soft drinks, or energy drinks, and cutting your sugar intake will also help you get more rest.

Quick Tips: Good Sleep Habits

The following tips about sleeping to strengthen your immune system make sense for all ages:

- Go to bed and awake at the same time each day, even on weekends. There is no way to make up for "lost sleep."

- Establish a daily "cool-down" time. One hour before bedtime dim the lights and eliminate noise. Use this time for low-level stimulation activities such as listening to quiet music or reading non-stimulating material.

- Associate beds with resting only. Talk on the phone or scan the Internet elsewhere.

- Don't drink caffeinated drinks in the afternoon or evening. Caffeine's stimulating effects will peak two to four hours after consumption, but they can linger in the body for several hours.

- Don't eat dinner close to bedtime, and don't overeat. Sleep can be disrupted by digestive systems working extra hard after a heavy meal. Make your last meal of the day a light one.

- Avoid exercise close to bedtime. Physical activity late in the day can affect your body's ability to relax into a peaceful slumber.

Boosting the Immune System

Getting enough sleep is absolutely critical for maintaining a strong immune system. Lack of sleep causes a decline of natural killer cells. Deep sleep helps to strengthen the immune system and repair any tissue damage. In fact, colds, flu, and sinus infections tend to make you feel sleepy for a good reason. When the immune system is battling these germs and viruses, it produces chemicals called cytokines, which cause the body to feel tired and sleepy. Your body works to conserve energy so that the immune system can mount up an attack against the infection.

Unfortunately too many people work forty-plus hours a week; when they catch a cold, come down with the flu, or develop a sinus infection, they keep pushing themselves. Does that sound like you? When you keep pushing yourself at the very time your body is signaling you to sleep, you are undermining your immune system and sabotaging your health. God created principles of health within your body that you need to obey. Cheating your body again and again ultimately can cause disastrous consequences. Good sleep habits can help prevent you from coming down with colds or flu. However, if you contract a virus, make sure that you take time to rest so that your body can heal. Make it a priority to get seven to eight hours of rest each night.

Quick Tips: Natural Sleep Protocol

- Before bed take a warm Epsom salts bath with lavender oil added. This will relax your muscles and mind, promoting restful sleep.
- Try some Sleepy Time or chamomile tea sweetened with stevia extract before you go to bed.
- CalMax Powder, which is a highly absorbable calcium-magnesium supplement, will help you sleep through the night. Kava and passionflower are natural relaxers, along with valerian root; they help ease tension and cause you to feel sleepy.
- Carbohydrates can also help to induce sleep. Pasta for dinner with vegetables (no meat) is the way to go.
- You may snack on brown rice, banana, or warm milk with honey.
- Try 3 mg of melatonin on a temporary basis to help reset your biological clock.
- Consider exercise. It is a wonderful stress reliever, which will in turn lighten your mental load.

Rest is vital when you have a cold or the flu. And don't assume a bad case of the sniffles or frequent sneezing is necessarily a cold. It could be chronic sinusitis, the most common chronic disease in the United States and a condition that affects about forty million people. Studies reveal that the vast majority of individuals with chronic colds lasting longer than two weeks actually have a sinus infection.[1]

If you have suffered from a sinus infection, it was one of two types: acute or chronic sinusitis.

Acute sinusitis is usually triggered by a cold. Symptoms of acute sinusitis include a cold that lasts longer than two weeks, yellow or green nasal drainage, a fever, cough, postnasal drip, facial pressure—especially around the cheeks, eyes, or forehead—pain in the upper molars and swelling of the face. Some people experience loss of the sense of smell. There is a good possibility that your sinuses are infected if pain occurs after tapping your cheekbones, the area around the bridge of your nose, or your forehead just over the eyebrows.

Chronic sinusitis usually produces fewer symptoms than acute sinusitis. Symptoms include nasal congestion, postnasal drainage, sore throat, cough, low-grade fever, decreased sense of taste and smell, and cold symptoms such as a constant runny nose. These symptoms usually will interfere with your sleep. In 1999 a Mayo Clinic study found that an immune system response to fungus, rather than bacterial infection, is the cause of most cases of chronic sinusitis. These researchers studied two hundred ten patients with chronic sinusitis and found forty different kinds of fungus, including candida, in the mucus of 96 percent of the patients. However, in a control group of healthy volunteers, similar organisms were found as well. Therefore, researchers concluded the immune systems of those with chronic sinusitis reacted dramatically differently than those of healthy individuals.

The unusual immune reaction was determined to be responsible for the chronic pain, inflammation, and swelling of the mucous membranes associated with sinusitis. This is now actually termed "allergic fungal sinusitis." And again, it's an immune system response and not an allergy to the fungus that is the cause of chronic sinus infection.[2]

Quick Tips: For Sleep Disorders

If a lack of sleep is weakening you in the battle against colds and flu, testing neurotransmitters is the best way to determine if you have depletion in brain chemicals that could be causing the problem. Testing can be completed whether you are taking medications or not. You can determine if your neurotransmitters are out of balance by taking the Brain Wellness Programs Self Test. Just go to www.neurogistics.com and click "Get Started." Use the practitioner code SLEEP (all caps). You can order the program, which includes a urine in-home test that will yield a report on your neurotransmitter levels. You'll be given a customized protocol with guidelines for the right amino acids for you to take to help correct your imbalances. Or call 866-843-8935 for more information.

Chapter 4

LIMIT SUGAR INTAKE

WHEN IT COMES to winning the battle with colds and flu, one of the wisest precautions you can take is avoiding sugar. Certain foods can actually impair the immune system, sabotaging its effectiveness. Sugar is at the top of the list. Excessive sugar consumption has been shown to suppress the body's immune response by inhibiting the immune function. This starts just thirty minutes after consumption and lasts for more than five hours. While sugar gives you a temporary lift, it eventually brings you down lower than where you started. As little as 100 grams of any form of sugar can reduce the ability of your immune system's army to engulf and destroy invaders. Since food manufacturers add sugar to so many processed and other foods, it requires constant vigilance to avoid ingesting too much.

In order for your immune system to work at peak efficiency, it needs certain nutrients and foods to fuel all its different areas and functions. Yet, feeding your body sugar, along with highly processed carbohydrates, bad fats, and fried foods, is like sending a soldier into battle with a pocketknife and a BB gun. So if you feel a cold or virus attack coming on, don't reach for a bowl of ice cream or peach cobbler. Remember, sweet treats can be hazardous to your health. At the very time you should be eating very little, even going on a liquid fast, you will add to the problem.

In addition to the dangers sugar intake poses during cold and flu season, a year-round habit of consuming too much sugar on a daily basis may be setting you up for low blood sugar (hypoglycemia). Even small blood sugar fluctuations disturb a person's sense of well-being. Larger fluctuations caused by consuming too much sugar cause feelings of depression, anxiety, mood swings, fatigue, and even aggressive behavior. Some studies have shown that people suffering from depression had fewer symptoms when sugar was removed from their diets.

Symptoms of anxiety and depression closely parallel many of the

18

symptoms of hypoglycemia: rapid pulse, crying spells, heart palpitations, weakness, cold sweats, irritability, fatigue, nightmares, twitching, and poor concentration. If these symptoms are familiar to you, it is possible you are suffering from low blood sugar. To help restore normal blood sugar levels, you need to focus on eating more fiber and protein foods at each meal and cutting back on simple sugars. It is very important that you have a protein snack between meals to help keep your blood sugar levels stable all day long.

Quick Tips: Perils of Too Much Sugar

An overload of sugar can depress your immune system in the following ways:

Mental and emotional signs

- Difficulty concentrating, forgetfulness, or absentmindedness
- Lack of motivation, loss of enthusiasm for plans and projects
- Increasing instability, reflected in inconsistent thoughts and actions
- Moody personality changes with emotional outbursts
- Irritability, mood swings

Brain and body symptoms

- Anxiety and panic attacks
- Bulimia
- Candidiasis, chronic fatigue syndrome
- Diabetes or hypoglycemia
- Food addiction due to stress; B vitamins and minerals are lost as a result of experiencing stress
- Obesity
- Menopausal mood swings and unusually low energy

- High cholesterol and triglycerides, leading to risk of atherosclerosis
- Excessive food cravings, especially before menstruation
- Tooth decay and gum loss[1]

Eliminating Sugar

It is true that eliminating sugar or even limiting it will not be easy. But in order to build your body's immune defenses, you must curtail such consumption. By combining low-glycemic foods (high-fiber foods) and adding amino acid supplementation and nutritional supplements to help balance your blood sugar, you will also optimize brain biochemistry. You can take various dietary supplements to aid the transition away from sugar, such as chromium picolinate, a B-complex vitamin, vitamin C, an adrenal gland supplement, and a calcium-magnesium supplement. Try a protein shake each morning and use stevia extract as a sugar-balancing herbal sweetener.

While lowering your sugar will help you in the battle against colds and flu, it is also wise to make the effort to balance your blood sugar. Low blood sugar can predispose you to developing diabetes later in life. Diabetes occurs when the body does not properly utilize the sugar and carbohydrates you consume. Because of years of abuse the pancreas is no longer able to produce adequate insulin, which creates the condition of high blood sugar. This can be very dangerous: diabetes can lead to heart and kidney disease, stroke, blindness, hypertension, and even death.

If you feel you are addicted to sugar, as many Americans are, you may feel helpless to change your lifestyle so drastically as to eliminate sugar. However, it isn't as difficult as you may imagine. Sugar cravings increase because they deplete the body of necessary elements it needs. For example, people who consume too much simple sugar and who are under constant stress typically have low levels of chromium. Taking a chromium supplement will help you wean yourself off simple sugars that have been robbing you of your health. One health expert has noticed her clients experiencing a heightened sense of well-being after following a healthy eating plan and taking chromium picolinate. Adding chromium to the diet seems to increase energy levels as well; clients noticed a more evenly sustained energy level.

Sugar Substitutes

In place of sugar, you can learn to use natural whole-food sweeteners, such as:

- Honey, a whole food, is twice as sweet as sugar and contains vitamins and enzymes (avoid if you are diabetic or have candida or low blood sugar).

- Rice syrup, made from rice and sugar, is 40 percent as sweet as sugar.

- Sucarat is a natural sweetener made from sugar cane juice. A concentrated sweetener, like honey, it should be used with caution if you have a blood sugar imbalance.

- Stevia is a natural sweetener that comes from South America and can be used in beverages, baking, and cooking. It is safe for those with blood sugar imbalances and/or candida and diabetes. Stevia comes in two forms, a liquid extract and a white powered extract.

- Fructose is a natural sweetener derived from fruit. It is twice as sweet as sugar; avoid if you have candida.

These natural sweeteners are noncaloric and safe for diabetics and hypoglycemics. What isn't safe are artificial sweeteners. In recent times America has jumped on the artificial sweetener bandwagon, thanks to our obsession and preoccupation with obesity. Although artificial sweeteners may seem like the solution for watching sugar calories, these "fake sugars" contain toxic and harmful ingredients that can damage our health. For instance, did you know that one of the components of aspartame is methanol—considered toxic even in small amounts? In addition, toxic levels of methanol have been associated with brain swelling, inflammation of the heart muscle and the pancreas, and even blindness! Simply put, aspartame is a synthetic chemical that can harm the body.

Chapter 5

SUPERFOODS THAT BUILD IMMUNITY

Your body is a tool needing proper care and feeding to enable you to achieve maximum potential in every area of life. So what you eat is a key component of avoiding colds and flu. Plus, a healthy diet will improve your quality of life, your mental and emotional state, and your spiritual well-being. A correct diet that includes superfoods gives you an edge. These foods will propel you to new highs that you never can achieve eating the standard Western meat-heavy, fat- and sugar-laden, carbohydrate-overloaded heavy diet. The typical diet contains all the things you want to avoid—animal and dairy products, sugar, fried foods, white flour, and refined foods. You may not be able to eliminate all of them, but strive to limit their consumption.

The best diet is a low-fat, high-fiber diet featuring whole grains, garlic, onions, fresh fruits, yogurt, and legumes. Cruciferous vegetables are healthy too. Examples are broccoli, cabbage, and Brussels sprouts, which contain indoles. These indoles help to protect breast tissue from estrogen metabolites (by-products of estrogen that can contribute to estrogen dominance). Superfoods cleanse and energize your body, and rapidly exit your system. The cleaner your body, the more you will radiate with good health.

Fantastic Fiber

Fiber is sorely lacking in most Americans' diets, yet this class of superfoods should be a part of everyone's daily regimen. It comes in two varieties: water soluble, which means it can dissolve in water, and the kind that is insoluble in water. Foods high in soluble fiber include oats, oat bran, guar gum, carrots, beans, apples, ground flaxseeds, psyllium, and citrus pectin. Foods high in insoluble fiber include wheat bran, most root vegetables, celery, and the skins of fruits.

Soluble fiber feeds the intestinal bacteria, especially the good bacteria. It also provides nourishment to the cells of the colon. Intestinal bacteria cause soluble fiber to ferment and form short-chain fatty acids. This, in turn, nourishes the cells of the large intestine. These short-chain fatty acids help to prevent the growth of yeast and harmful bacteria. Soluble fiber helps to lower cholesterol, control blood sugar, and create a sensation of fullness so that you will be less likely to overeat. However, if you eat too much soluble fiber, such as too many beans or too much guar gum, you can develop an overgrowth of intestinal bacteria—not to mention excessive bloating, gas, and abdominal discomfort. There's a reason for the saying that you should do everything in moderation.

Insoluble fiber inactivates many intestinal toxins. It also helps to prevent harmful bacteria and parasites from attaching themselves to the wall of your intestines by acting like a sweeping broom. Since both forms of fiber are beneficial, it is wise to eat food that contains a mixture of soluble and insoluble fibers. Rice bran, oat bran, legumes (such as beans and peas), apples, pears, and berries contain both sources of fiber.

Green Superfoods

One of the most effective tools for building health is found in the class of foods called green superfoods. Supercharged with nutrition, they are like receiving a small transfusion to enhance immunity and promote energy. One of the richest sources of many essential nutrients, they are nutritionally more concentrated and potent than regular greens like salads and green vegetables. In addition, green superfoods are purposely grown and harvested to maximize and ensure high vitamin, mineral, and amino acid concentrations. Some examples:

- Blue and blue-green algae are the most potent source of beta carotene available in the world. They are brimming with superior quality proteins, fiber, vitamins, minerals, and enzymes.

- Spirulina is extremely high in protein and rich in B vitamins, amino acids, beta-carotene, and essential fatty acids. Easy to digest, spirulina boosts energy quickly and sustains it.

- Barley grass contains vitamins, minerals, proteins, enzymes, and chlorophyll. It contains more calcium, vitamin C, and vitamin B$_{12}$ than cow's milk. And it helps inflammatory conditions of the stomach and digestive system.

+ Wheatgrass has been used worldwide for many serious diseases to rebuild, cleanse, and strengthen the body because of its incredible nutritional value.

+ Kyo-Green by Wakunaga of America contains barley, wheatgrass, chlorella, and kelp. This is a potent formula that helps cleanse the bloodstream, detoxify the system, and supply the body with minerals, enzymes, and many important nutrients.

These green superfoods are also high in flavonoids, which gives them anti-inflammatory, antitumor, and antiviral effects.

In addition to superfoods, greens such as spinach, collard greens, beet greens, cilantro, and parsley are high in chlorophyllin. Chlorophyllins fight cancer by inhibiting many different carcinogens. Chlorophyllin can help reduce cancer-causing substances, called heterocyclic amines (HCAs), in cooked meats and fried foods. They help reduce the carcinogens in cigarette smoke and protect DNA from radiation damage. Not only are green foods packed with this vital substance, but also their magnesium levels give them a double punch. Magnesium helps to cleanse the GI tract. High-chlorophyll foods are effective virus fighters, making them quite useful in cold and flu season.

CRUCIFEROUS VEGETABLES

Mentioned earlier, these healthy vegetables are cancer blasters. Vegetables such as cabbage, brussels sprouts, cauliflower, broccoli, kale, collard greens, mustard greens, watercress, turnips, and radishes contain more phytonutrients with anticancer properties than any other family of vegetables. The word *cruciferous* comes from the same word root as *crucifying*, which means "to place one on a cross." Oddly, the flowers of cruciferous vegetables contain two components that appear similar to the shape of a cross.

The potent cancer-fighting phytonutrients in the cruciferous vegetables family include indoles, isothiocyanates, and sulforaphanes, which are sulfur-containing compounds. They also contain phenols, coumarins, dithiolthiones, and glucosinolates, as well as other phytonutrients that are yet to be discovered. Indoles, especially indole-3-carbinol, are potent cancer antagonists. Sulforaphanes stimulate liver detoxification enzymes. Isothiocyanates induce production of detoxification enzymes by the liver, and they prevent damage to the DNA. Studies have correlated a high intake of cruciferous vegetables, especially cabbage—with lower rates of cancers, especially cancers of the breast and colon.[1] While you may be cancer free today, remember good health is a holistic picture. You should arm yourself against all disease, short- and long-term.

With these cruciferous veggies, broccoli sprouts have the highest concentration of the protective phytonutrients. Select young broccoli sprouts that are about three days old. They contain twenty to fifty times more of the potent phytonutrient sulforaphane than mature broccoli. Juicing cruciferous vegetables on a regular basis can help your liver to detoxify from pesticides, chemicals, drugs, and other pollutants.

Mighty Mushrooms

One of the strongest superfoods is also one of the smallest. Mushrooms are deserving of the label, though. Researchers have discovered that certain types of "power mushrooms" are filled with a grocery list of substances that may help in fighting disease. The most exciting report is that they boost immunity, a valuable component in reaching your good health goals. Mushrooms produce many beneficial compounds that help their survival against other fungi and microbes.[2]

The same substances that mushrooms use for defense can help humans as well. Mushrooms contain compounds known as polysaccharides. Polysaccharides spark the immune system by helping the body to create T-cells, which are immune system warriors in our bodies that destroy invaders. Incorporating any of the power mushrooms into your diet helps create a synergism within your immune system. Here are three of these power-packed varieties:

+ Reishi, which stimulates immunity, has antitumor properties, is an anti-inflammatory, and helps to alleviate arthritis.

+ Shiitake has possible antiviral, anticancer properties and is an energizer. It is also delicious when used in cooking.

+ Maitake has antitumor properties. It may also protect the liver and lower blood pressure. It contains beta-glucans, which are chemicals that boost immunity.[3]

Quick Tips: Healing Power of Coconuts

One of the most amazing superfoods around, coconuts can help strengthen you against colds and flu. Coconuts will help your body fight off infection—the body converts it to monolaurin, which fights off infections (viral or bacterial). Coconut water makes a fantastic water base for natural shakes and raw drinks; it is the most complete hydrating liquid a human can consume. With the exception of B_6 and B_{12}, the water and flesh from young coconuts contains the full range of B vitamins. Since they break down carbohydrates and proteins, these are essential for providing energy. They also support nervous system function.

Coconut water is a natural isotonic beverage. It is more hydrating than water or any electrolyte sports drink since it only hydrates you while cooling down body temperature and providing energy. You can buy all natural and canned varieties to take with you on trips. Coconut is also a potent antibacterial and antifungal agent. It is a great cleaner of our gut and is something that can help heal the gut, should problems like leaky gut syndrome occur.

Other Superfoods

Ginger

This spice quickens and sharpens the senses and boosts memory. Ginger helps combat nausea, motion sickness, and vomiting. It is good for indigestion because it absorbs excess stomach acid, is useful for circulatory problems, and is an antioxidant. However, ginger is a circulatory stimulant, so consult your physician or health advisor if you have a heart condition or other condition that could be affected by its use.

Ellagic acid

Ellagic acid is found in strawberries, raspberries, grapes, and black currants. This powerful healing substance has been shown to inhibit cancer that has been chemically induced in rats.[4] Ellagic acid also protects against damage by toxins to chromosomes, which are our genetic blueprint. Finally, ellagic acid is a powerful antioxidant.

Chamomile tea

Chamomile tea benefits digestion and also has calming properties. It is an excellent tea to drink after dinner to help calm you before going to bed.

Healthy Juices

Here are four recipes that will strengthen your immune system while filling you with pep for the day. With all of these, juice and add more ice or water if desired. Add 1–3 tablespoons of the pulp back to the juice and stir.

Recipe: Green Limeade

1 package organic field greens—red, green, or romaine (not iceberg)
6 organic limes, peeled (if blended in a Vitamix, use 1/8 of the peel)
1 small piece of ginger
2 organic apples
1 bunch organic celery
1 organic cucumber

Recipe: Vegetable Cocktail

5 organic carrots

1 organic green pepper

1 organic broccoli stalk

2 stalks organic celery

1 organic cucumber

1 organic hot pepper

1 organic lemon

Recipe: Spinach Pineapple Drink

1 bag organic spinach

1 organic pineapple, skin cut off

1 bunch organic celery

4 organic cucumbers

2 organic lemons, peeled

Recipe: Vitamix Drink

3-4 organic baby carrots or handful of organic dandelion leaf, organic spinach, organic kale, or organic collard greens

1/8 organic lime with skin or 1/8 organic lemon with skin

1 organic Granny Smith apple or 4 ounces organic blueberries, organic blackberries, organic strawberries, or organic raspberries

Handful of organic broccoli, organic cauliflower, organic cabbage, organic watercress, or organic beets

1-2 stalks organic celery (optional)

4 ounces water

4 ounces ice

You can vary your Vitamix drink by making different selections from the four main groups. It is best to rotate fruits and veggies over four days. For example, one day use carrots, lime, blueberries, and broccoli; and the next day use spinach, lemon, Granny Smith apples, and watercress.

Chapter 6

HOME REMEDIES FOR COLDS AND FLU RELIEF

WHEN THE NEXT cold and flu season arrives, stop running to the pharmacy at the first sign of symptoms. There are many natural remedies that can help you beat the symptoms of a cold, flu, or sinus infection after you have already become ill. Natural foods and home remedies work as effectively as over-the-counter and prescription medications but without any adverse side effects.

Recipe for Flu and Cold Medicine

While influenza and colds are common, avoid running to the pharmacy if they appear. Raw natural foods act as a potent source of healing without any side effects. Drink the following blend on an empty stomach three times a day, replacing meals for a few days. Or try it while fasting for at least twenty-four hours and see how quickly you heal.

- Four oranges: Peel oranges but keep the white pith. Oranges and papayas are an excellent antioxidant.
- One papaya: Skin the fruit and remove all seeds. Both oranges and papayas will cleanse toxicity, which is what leads to a weakened immune system. They also help cleanse your intestinal tract. They are full of calcium and rich in vitamin A, beta-carotene, and vitamin C.
- Six figs: Take off the stem and make sure they are soft. These are one of the best mucus dissolvers.
- Optional: one hot pepper, jalapeño, or orange habanero pepper to cleanse the sinus cavities and fight bacteria. Hot peppers contain phytoantibiotics, which wipe out bacteria-causing sickness.

- Optional: one avocado for added thickness to offset the hot peppers.

For example, raw foods represent medicine for the body and provide incredible levels of energy, health, and vitality. When coming down with a sore throat that may signal a cold or flu, stop eating solid food and ingest only healthy foods. The following can be liquefied in a blender or juicer to provide an assortment of rapid immune system boosts:

+ One ripe orange habanero pepper (or a ripe jalapeno): You will feel this cleanse you as fire-like sensations course through your body, killing bacteria and viruses. It also will start to clear out nasal passages of mucus almost immediately.

+ Two cloves of garlic and one slice of ginger: Garlic and ginger are natural antibiotics that boost a weakened immune system. Ginger also helps reduce swelling in the throat. These are "power twins" for fighting infections.

+ Six figs: Figs are amazing at dissolving mucus and cleansing the gastrointestinal tract helping to detox your body.

+ A handful of parsley or kale: Both of these are rich in iron, which builds strong red-blood corpuscles.

+ Two organic apples (or four organic pears): Apples and pears contain pectin that helps to remove toxins. They help with bowel movements, which drains the lymphatic system and alleviates swelling in a sore throat and tonsils.

+ One ounce organic, cold-pressed, extra-virgin olive oil: Olive oil helps to build strong white blood corpuscles.

Natural Beverages

Drinking tea may sound like a hocus-pocus method for fighting infectious diseases, but that isn't the case. For example, goldenseal can be used to make a tea that will address respiratory problems and sinusitis, two ailments that may accompany colds and flu. Goldenseal may fight certain bacterial and parasitic infections, but it should not be taken for long periods of time (two weeks at a time maximum). A proper dosage is a cup of tea (2–4 grams) three times daily, or if using a tincture, taking 1½–3 teaspoons three times daily.

Ever hear of elderberry? Native Americans used tea made from elderberry flowers to treat respiratory infections. Elderberry extract contains a high percentage of three flavonoids that have been shown to have antiviral properties. A study published in the *Journal of Alternative and Complementary Medicine* in 1995 examined the flu-fighting capabilities of Sambucol, which is an elderberry extract preparation. The study found that elderberry interfered with the growth of multiple strains of influenza A and B viruses in cell cultures.[1]

During a flu outbreak in an Israeli kibbutz, twenty-seven subjects were given either elderberry or a placebo for three days. The results were amazing: 90 percent of those taking elderberry were completely cured within three days, while most of those who took the placebo needed six days to recover.[2] You can brew a tea with this amazing plant or take 2–4 tablespoons a day of a standardized extract (or as directed by your physician).

Here is a recipe for another healing tea that is good for fighting a sore throat, cold, flu, and infections. The following makes one serving:

Recipe: Healing Tea
_____

> 2-inch piece fresh ginger root, juiced
>
> Juice of 1/2 medium lemon
>
> 2 cups purified water
>
> 1 tablespoon loose licorice tea, or 1 licorice herbal tea bag (optional)

> 4-5 whole cloves
>
> 1 stick cinnamon, broken
>
> Dash cardamom
>
> Dash nutmeg

> Place all ingredients in a saucepan and simmer for about 10 minutes. Strain and drink while warm.

Another cold-busting beverage includes grapefruit, which is loaded with vitamin C and bioflavonoids, especially in the white pithy part. These nutrients support the immune cells. You can also use carrots, which are rich in beta-carotene, another immune cell superfood. Fresh ginger root is loaded with zinc, which is vital for the immune system; in Chinese medicine, it is used for treating colds. Cayenne pepper acts as a decongestant and expectorant. Drink your cold away with this recipe (one serving):

Recipe: Cold Buster

> 1 grapefruit, peeled
>
> 1 carrot, green top removed, ends trimmed, scrubbed, and juiced
>
> 2-3 kale leaves
>
> 1-inch chunk ginger root, juiced
>
> Dash of cayenne pepper

> Cut produce to fit your juicer's feed tube. Juice ingredients and stir. Pour into a glass and drink as soon as possible.

For cold or flu sufferers who are also dealing with clogged sinuses, radish juice is a traditional remedy to open up the sinuses and support mucous membranes. This simple recipe also makes one serving:

Recipe: Sinus Solution

> 2 vine-ripened tomatoes
>
> 1/2 cucumber, peeled if not organic
>
> 6 radishes with green leaves
>
> 1/2 lime, peeled if not organic

Cut produce to fit your juicer's feed tube. Juice ingredients and stir. Pour into a glass and drink as soon as possible.

The Natural Way

Herbs and various natural methods are another effective treatment in treatment of colds and flu. One in particular that has become popular in recent years in the United States is echinacea. Historically, Native Americans commonly used echinacea as a medicinal herb. Although American doctors picked up on it, its use faded in the late 1800s. In the 1930s German doctors rediscovered it, and it has remained popular overseas since that time.

There are three different species of the plant: *E. angustifolia*, *E. purpurea*, and *E. pallida*. Germany's Commission E, the government agency charged with investigating herbs, recommends treating colds with *E. purpurea*. Although it boosts the immune system's response to colds, flu, and other infections, echinacea is most commonly used in the treatment of the common cold. Start taking it as soon as you notice any cold symptoms. Take echinacea in 200 milligram (mg) doses three times a day for three weeks, followed by one week off for best results. Generally speaking, you should take echinacea the same way as you would take an antibiotic.

However, don't take echinacea if you are allergic to ragweed or if you have an autoimmune disease, such as lupus, rheumatoid arthritis, multiple sclerosis, or any other autoimmune disease. Also, do not take echinacea if you are pregnant.

Here are some home remedies that are useful for the effects of colds and flu.

Recipe: Flu Fighter

1 handful watercress or parsley

1 dark green lettuce leaf

1 turnip, scrubbed, ends trimmed, you can include leaves

3 carrots, scrubbed well, tops removed, ends trimmed

1–2 garlic cloves (garlic is nature's natural antibiotic)

1/2 lemon, peeled if not organic

1/2 green apple such as Granny Smith or pippin

Bunch up watercress or parsley and wrap in lettuce leaf. Cut produce to fit your juicer's feed tube. Push lettuce wrap through slowly, and follow with the remaining ingredients. Stir the juice, pour into a glass, and drink as soon as possible.

THREE RECIPES FOR HEALING A SORE THROAT

Recipe #1:

6–8 ounces of warm water (preferably fresh spring water)

The juice of a 1/2 lemon

A few cut-up pieces of fresh raw ginger or 1 tablespoon of ginger powder

1 teaspoon or tablespoon of raw honey

Recipe #2:

Create a ginger tea by simmering three to four slices of fresh ginger in a cup of water for six to eight minutes.

Recipe #3:

4 lemons

Several slices ginger root

Stevia to taste

Juice lemons, then scrub well and peel. Slice thinly, and add to the juice. Add ginger root. Cover all with plenty of boiling water; cover and steep until cool. Strain off the liquid, and add stevia and additional water to taste. Drink hot.[3]

If dealing with a cold at the same time, apply a ginger and cayenne compress to the chest to help loosen mucus.

NATURAL COUGH SYRUP

You can make your own cough syrup from six onions, ½ cup honey, and a pinch of cayenne pepper. Cook in a saucepan on low heat for about two hours. Strain the mixture to remove the onions. Take 1 tablespoon every two to three hours as needed.

Chapter 7

VITAMINS

THE "NATURAL" HEDGE of protection inside the human body known as the immune system protects us from a vast onslaught of diseases and illnesses. This incredible system protects you from everything from the sniffles of a cold to the destruction of cancer. An overreactive immune system can attack our own body's cells, resulting in diseases such as lupus and rheumatoid arthritis (autoimmune diseases). A failure of the immune system can result in cancer, and an overly sensitive immune system can result in allergies. A weakened immune system accelerates the aging process.

To maintain your immune system's fighting edge, your body needs to maintain a good, steady supply of basic vitamins and minerals. Today's modern diet does not always provide the essentials. In fact, even if your diet is rich with fruits and vegetables, there is a good chance they were grown in depleted soil. Certain vitamins and minerals are critically important for your immune system to function at peak efficiency, which is vital during cold and flu season.

Therefore, to maintain the strength and power of your immune system, take a comprehensive multivitamin-mineral supplement every day. A comprehensive multivitamin is important to provide the basic vitamins and minerals for your body that it cannot make for itself.

Essential Vitamins

A high-quality multiple vitamin contains vitamins, minerals, and most of the antioxidants your body requires on a daily basis. However, shop with care. The trend toward genetically modified foods (GMO) has even hit vitamin production. These supplements may be genetically modified. For example, vitamin C is often made from corn. Vitamin E is usually made from soy. Vitamins A, B_2, B_6, B_{12}, D, and K may have fillers derived from GMO corn sources, such as starch, glucose, and maltodextrin.[1]

Currently, labeling of GMO food is not required; therefore, you must carefully examine labels of packaged products to see if they contain corn flour or cornmeal, soy flour, cornstarch, textured vegetable protein, corn syrup, or modified food starch. Check labels of soy sauce, tofu, soy beverages, soy protein isolate, soy milk, soy ice cream, margarine, and soy lecithin, among dozens of other products. If it doesn't specify organic or non-GMO, the chances are strong that they are GMO foods.

Quick Tips: Choosing a Multivitamin

When choosing a multivitamin, it is important to remember that not all vitamins are created equal. Here are some considerations for helping you to make the best choices:

- Look for the "USP" number on the label. This number gives you the percentage of the product that has been formulated to dissolve after one hour in bodily fluids. The percentage should be as high as possible and will vary from product to product.

- Make sure the iron in your multivitamin is either ferrous fumarate or ferrous sulfate because they are the most absorbable forms.

- For best absorption, take your multivitamin with meals and not on an empty stomach. Otherwise you may experience nausea.

- Another important tip is to make sure that you take your multivitamin with a meal that contains a little fat. Fat-soluble vitamins (A, D, and E) need a little fat to get inside your system and go to work.

Once you have found a safe multivitamin source, what are the essential vitamins it contains? They start with the first letter of the alphabet. If your body lacks enough vitamin A, you will tend to be prone to many types of infections, especially colds and flu. Vitamin A works to maintain the structural integrity of the mucous membranes. It is also vitally important in the production of T-cells. A deficiency of vitamin A will cause your thymus gland to shrink, resulting in an impaired immune system. Many physicians are concerned about vitamin A overdosing, since it's associated with liver damage, loss of hair, headaches, vomiting, and other symptoms. Yet vitamin A overdosing is extremely rare; inadequate consumption of vitamin A is common. Approximately 5,000 to 10,000 IU of vitamin A daily is a safe dosage, although pregnant women should limit use to 5,000 IU per day.

Some people believe they don't need vitamin A because they take supplements of beta-carotene. They reason that since beta-carotene is a precursor to vitamin A, it's all they really need. However, vitamin A, beta-carotene, and other carotenoids all have independent roles to play in strengthening and protecting immunity. Therefore, all of these nutrients should be taken regularly. Vitamin A is present in most multivitamins.

B-complex vitamins are also very important for optimal immune function. Vitamin B_5, or pantothenic acid, is important for maintaining a healthy thymus gland and for antibody production. Folic acid is important for optimal function of T-cells and B-cells, as is vitamin B_6. Vitamin B_{12} is needed by phagocytes to kill bacteria. A comprehensive multivitamin should have adequate doses of B complex.

Vitamin C is also extremely important for the immune system; it is both an antiviral and antibacterial agent. Vitamin C strengthens connective tissue and also neutralizes toxic substances that are released from phagocytes.

In 1970 Dr. Linus Pauling released the book *Vitamin C and the Common Cold*.[2] He was one of the most prominent and respected scientists of the twentieth century and had been awarded two Nobel Prizes. But he stirred up tremendous controversy in the medical community when he recommended that people take 1,000 to 2,000 mg of vitamin C daily for general well-being. To fight a cold, he recommended upping the dosage to 4,000 to 10,000 mg a day.

Dr. Pauling found that supplementing with 1,000 mg of vitamin C daily reduced the incidence of colds by 45 percent and reduced cold symptoms by 63 percent.[3] Best-selling author and health expert Dr. Don Colbert recommends a preventive dose of 1,000 mg of vitamin C taken daily, preferably 250 mg three to four times a day or 500 mg twice a day. In case of a cold or sinus infection, he suggests boosting this to 2,000 mg a day, preferably in powdered form, every two to three hours. Maintain this dosage for several days, and then gradually taper off until you're back to 1,000 mg a day as a maintenance dose. However, consult with your physician before starting a high-dose vitamin C therapy.

Vitamin E is another essential vitamin that helps to preserve and strengthen the immune system function. A weakened immune system can be helped by taking vitamin E in natural form, using a dosage of 800 IU daily. A multiple vitamin may not contain the full recommended daily allowance of vitamin E, so check the panel for further information.

Folic acid is contained in many multiple vitamins; one of the most common nutritional deficiencies in the world is of folic acid. Part of the reason is we simply don't eat enough vegetables. In addition, some medications, such as birth control pills, contribute to this deficiency. Alcohol and stress can play a part also.

Adequate folic acid is vital to good health; without it we stand to increase our risk of heart disease by having elevated levels of homocysteine (a toxic amino acid). Folic acid is necessary for DNA repair, and it keeps your immune system strong. Studies have shown that high doses of folic acid can eliminate most of the precancerous cells on women with cervical dysplasia.[4] However, pregnant women should be wary of taking folic acid and consult their doctor about this issue.

Natural Substances

Although supplements are part of a good health regimen, remember to not rely solely on this form of arming yourself in the battle against viruses. Science is discovering a fascinating array of natural substances that strengthen the immune system, including substances in the plant kingdom. Researchers have identified many substances that can strengthen the immune system, as well as decrease the occurrence of many forms of cancer and heart disease. One such group is known as antioxidants. These include vitamin C, vitamin E, beta-carotene, and selenium.

There are many different food sources for the antioxidants we need. You can get plenty of vitamins C and E and beta-carotene from yellow, orange, and dark green fruits and vegetables. Almonds (about ten per day) can supply vitamin E.

Here are some other food sources:

+ Vitamin C—bell peppers, citrus fruits, strawberries, cantaloupe, broccoli, cauliflower, potatoes, tomatoes, other fruits, and dark leafy greens, such as spinach, kale, and mustard greens

+ Vitamin E—vegetable oils (olive, canola), wheat germ, wholegrain bread and pasta

+ Beta-carotene—broccoli, cantaloupe, carrots, spinach, squash, pumpkin, sweet potatoes, apricots, and other dark green, orange, and yellow vegetables

Celery is another potent natural source of fighting infections. Especially healthy for your skin because it cleans the cells and remove dirt skin oils, among its other benefits are promoting the proper functioning of the immune system. What's more, celery provides your body vitamin A and is a great source of B vitamins, such as B_1, B_2, and B_6.

Avocados are rich in potassium (60 percent more than bananas), vitamin A, vitamin E, and B vitamins. Besides helping you fight colds, the oil from avocados aids in triggering the production of collagens. So incorporating more avocados into your diet will mean less wrinkles and a more even, toned skin appearance. The brighter the fruit, the more beta-carotene they contain, so look for vibrant green ones that are slightly soft to the touch.

Chapter 8

MINERALS

J UST AS YOUR body needs certain vitamins to strengthen your immune system, minerals are also vitally important for proper functioning. Mineral deficiencies are even more common in the standard American diet than vitamin deficiencies; it is common for women to get too little iron and calcium in their diets. Minerals will help build, strengthen, and heal your body. Every living cell depends on minerals for proper function and structure. The balance of your body depends upon proper levels and ratios of different minerals. Minerals are crucial for proper nerve function, regulation of muscle tone, formation of blood and bone, and composition of body fluids. The entire cardiovascular system relies heavily on proper mineral balance.

To give you an idea of how minerals boost your health, here are several examples of just some of their benefits:

- Calcium: Provides strong bones, teeth, and muscle and nerve function; aids in blood clotting
- Chloride: Aids digestion; works with sodium to maintain fluid balance
- Chromium: Provides proper carbohydrate metabolism
- Copper: Aids in formation of blood cells and connective tissues
- Iodine: Maintains proper thyroid function
- Manganese: Aids calcium, phosphorous, and magnesium metabolism; provides essential support for healthy bones

Even though you can get minerals from some food sources, it is sometimes necessary to use mineral supplements to obtain sufficient amounts for your body's needs. Here is where a multiple vitamin plays a crucial role in strengthening your body since it contains minerals as well as vitamins. As mentioned in chapter 7, a daily multiple vitamin is a basic ingredient in a good health regimen. One reason is that it contains trace amounts of minerals that are vital to the functioning of your immune system.

Why is it necessary to take a multiple vitamin and other supplements? The outdated theory of mainstream medicine that holds that you can get all of the vitamins and minerals you need from your diet is slowly dying out. More and more physicians realize that, while it may have been true that your grandparents received all the nutrition they required from their foods, this is simply not the case in the modern generation. Mineral-depleted soils and chemical agribusiness farming and marketing methods almost guarantee that you will not get anywhere near the ideal nutritional value that you need for health from the foods you buy at most supermarkets.

Instead of nourishing your body, traditionally grown and processed, "devitalized" food actually abuses your body. When foods have been grown in nutrient-poor soil, they may look pretty, but that's about all. When our soil has been robbed of important minerals and nutrients, the food it produces will be nutritionally poor as well.

Magnificent Minerals

One of the minerals in a multiple vitamin is selenium, which is important for building and maintaining superior immunity. Selenium deficiency causes a reduction in T-cell activity and antibody production. It can also lower your resistance to developing viral and bacterial infections. Selenium supplements significantly enhance the body's production of white blood cells—especially T-cells and natural killer cells. You should take approximately 200 micrograms (mcg) of selenium a day; check the information panel on your multivitamin for the dosage it includes.

Zinc is another element and is important for the immune system. In fact, it's the most important mineral to the thymus gland. Zinc is required for cell-mediated immunity. A deficiency in zinc will cause a decrease in T-cells, natural killer cells, and thymic hormone; in addition, zinc has been found to prevent cold viruses from reproducing themselves. However, too much can cause harmful effects; 15 to 30 mg daily is sufficient (the amount found in most multiple vitamins).

A study on zinc throat lozenges found that when subjects who were developing cold symptoms dissolved zinc lozenges in their mouths every two hours, they recovered much faster.[1] Those who took the lozenges recovered in an average of 4.4 days compared with 7.6 days for those who were given a placebo.

Most American diets are low in zinc. Some experts believe our low zinc intake is the reason so many of us have immune problems. Nevertheless, all zinc is not equal. Zinc gluconate or zinc acetate is preferred to zinc picolinate or zinc citrate. Make sure that your zinc throat lozenges do not contain sugar, citrate, or tartrate fillers, since zinc binds to these fillers and becomes less available. Zinc is also available in a nasal gel called Zicam. Research suggests that the length and severity of a cold may be cut in half when treated with zinc nasal spray within two days of the onset of symptoms. Whether you elect to use zinc nose spray or zinc throat lozenges, it's important that you begin within twenty-four hours of the first sign of symptoms for the maximum benefit.

Your body also needs between 300–400 mg of magnesium a day. Americans commonly don't get enough magnesium in their diets. Although most multivitamins only provide a portion of the recommended daily allowance, you should be able to get the rest you need through eating a varied diet with green vegetables and whole grains.

Magnesium is a cofactor used in more than three hundred different enzyme reactions. Magnesium also helps to manufacture DNA for protein synthesis, fatty acid synthesis, and removal of toxic substances. Therefore, it is critically important for the liver to have adequate amounts of magnesium so that the liver can continue to perform its other roles of protein, carbohydrate, and fat metabolism.

Other Steps

In addition to a multivitamin, there are other healthy supplements and substances that you can take that either contain minerals or move them around.

Eat royal jelly (2 teaspoons daily)

This jelly is known to be a blessing for the body against asthma, liver disease, skin disorders, and immune suppression. This is because it is rich in vitamins, minerals, enzymes, and hormones. In addition, it possesses antibiotic and antibacterial properties. It is interesting to note that it naturally contains a high concentration of pantothenic acid.

Drink pure water

While you likely rarely think of water's mineral capacity, this should be a daily priority. First of all, it helps keep you hydrated and helps all of your body's systems to work more efficiently. In addition, water promotes proper elimination, removes toxins, and lessens arthritic pain. It also helps to transport proteins, vitamins, minerals, and sugars for assimilation. Water helps the body work at its peak.

Enjoy fresh fruits and vegetables

These foods are enzyme rich and full of vitamins, minerals, and fiber. They are also packed with phytonutrients and antioxidants that prevent cancer, heart disease, strokes, osteoporosis, and most other degenerative diseases.

Try juicing

In addition to water and easily absorbed protein and carbohydrates, juice provides essential fatty acids, vitamins, minerals, enzymes, and phytonutrients. Fresh juice is loaded with minerals. There are about two dozen minerals that your body needs to function well. Minerals, along with vitamins, are components of enzymes. They make up part of bone, teeth, and blood tissue, and they help maintain normal cellular function.

Minerals occur in inorganic forms in the soil, and plants incorporate them into their tissues. As a part of this process, the minerals are combined with organic molecules into easily absorbable forms, which makes plant food an excellent dietary source of minerals. Juicing is believed to provide even better mineral absorption than whole vegetables because the process of juicing liberates minerals into a highly absorbable, easily digestible form.

Eat organic

Organic foods promote good health because they are in their raw, natural state. They are not sprayed with pesticides, chemicals, fungicides, or other harmful substances. Organically grown food also has much lower quantities of toxic trace minerals, such as lead, mercury, and aluminum. Plus, various studies have shown that organic food contains much more iron, potassium, magnesium, and calcium than conventional crops. Most studies show organic food has up to ten times the mineral content of conventional foods.

Typical diets that include processed foods—white flour, sugar, coffee, and soft drinks—cause a pH imbalance in the body and become too acidic. Too much acid in one's body will decrease the body's ability to absorb nutrients and minerals, decrease the energy production in cells, and make the body more susceptible to illness and fatigue. Therefore, maintaining a healthy pH balance is necessary for optimal health.

Chapter 9

SUPPLEMENTS

Since good health is a holistic picture, before we review some supplements that will help your immune system, a word about eating healthy: taking vitamins and other nutrients while continuing to eat poorly is similar to never changing the oil or oil filter in your car and yet continuing to drive it. Periodically you might add small amounts of oil to the car to keep the oil level in normal range. This is, in essence, what most people are doing in their mistaken belief that they can continue to eat junk food, yet take a vitamin a day or multitudes of vitamins and be healthy. Some of the people who take the longest list of supplements are also the sickest—because they follow a poor diet.

Most chronic diseases, such as heart disease, diabetes, arthritis, and cancer, are usually associated with nutritional deficiencies. However, dieting and eating too much sugar, fats, processed foods, fast foods, and other devitalized and inflammatory foods will literally drain the life out of you. They will constipate you, make your tissues acidic, introduce toxins into your system, inflame your tissues, drain you of nutrient reserves, and accelerate degeneration. Americans have been duped into believing that they can continue to eat whatever they want and that simply taking a vitamin, or a multitude of vitamins and supplements, can magically neutralize or protect themselves from their junk-filled diets. Not true!

Quick Tips: Supplement Support for the Common Cold

- Vitamin C: 3,000 mg
- Grapefruit seed extract capsules
- Echinacea
- Ginger compress on chest
- White flower oil on throat area, neck, and chest

- NutriBiotic Nasal Spray
- NAC (N-acetyl cysteine)
- Kyolic Garlic: six capsules daily
- Goldenseal
- Beta-glucan

However, the good news is that when you improve your eating plan and starting consuming more fruits, vegetables, and organic meats, your body will notice. When the quality of the food coming in is of higher quality than what you used to consume, your body begins to discard the lower grade materials to make room for new, superior materials. The amazing human body will always choose the best materials you give it to make new and healthier tissue. The body always tries to produce health—and always succeeds unless you interfere with the process. This self-curing nature of the body is evident in many conditions such as the common cold, fevers, cuts, swellings, and bruises.

Still, as we pointed out in the last two chapters on vitamins and minerals, you can't always get the nutritional boost you need from food. Proper supplements can help strengthen your immunity and make you less prone to sickness. Here are some supplements to undergird your body's defense system.

Healthy Supplements

Coenzyme Q_{10}

Coenzyme Q_{10} is a necessary component of cellular energy production and respiration. It enhances energy levels in every cell of the body, providing increased energy and exercise tolerance and optimal nutritional support of the cardiovascular system. It is especially supportive of tissues that require a lot of energy, such as periodontal tissue, the heart muscle, and the cells of the body's defense system. The suggested dose is two to four capsules per day, with meals.

Olive leaf extract

Derived from the Mediterranean olive tree, olive leaf extract is popular in herbal and folk remedies and has benefited mankind for over one hundred fifty years. Oleuropein, the active nutrient in olive leaf, is a powerful foe against bacteria, fungi, parasites, and yeast. Olive leaf provides natural protection and a healthy environment for cells without suppressing immune system function or harming beneficial microflora. A suggested dose is one to two capsules of standardized extract (500 mg) per day, with meals.[1]

Melatonin

Produced by the pineal gland, melatonin is a hormone that regulates the body's wake/sleep/wake cycle. The hormone is secreted in a circadian rhythm by enzymes, which are activated by darkness and depressed by light. Nightly melatonin supplementation can boost the performance of immune systems that are compromised during sleep by age, drugs, or stress. The suggested dose is one 3-mg capsule, one-half to one hour before bedtime. (Caution: Do not take if you are pregnant or lactating.)

Colloidal silver

This dietary supplement is made of pure silver and distilled water. Throughout the centuries it fulfilled multiple functions. Hundreds of years ago, during the origins of the pharmaceutical market, people used natural products to prevent infections instead of turning to antibiotics, which have polluted our bodies and water (not to mention creating more "superbugs" that can prove nearly impossible to fight). Dating back much further in history, colloidal silver was a leading health product, due to its efficiency in supporting the immune system. With the expansion of the medical world—and, consequently, the pharmaceutical industry—its use did not increase. Yet, ironically, laboratories and specialists discovered new uses for this product, such as a stress reliever and skin conditioner, and for enhanced physical performance.

The rich concentration of silver molecules in colloidal silver essentially destroys bacteria and viruses and keeps the immune system safe and sound. Moreover, products based on colloidal silver are nontoxic.

Nor do they lose power to act when in contact with other antibiotics or medical treatments. The silver component has been proven to be compatible with the human body and no tolerance limit found to prevent its use.

Furthermore, unlike antibiotics medications, colloidal silver does not require long-term treatment. This happens because silver particles destroy viruses and germs from initial contact. Because of this, bacteria and other microorganisms do not have time to develop a firewall against these particles. With outbreaks of strange viruses occurring regularly, this is one of the best ways to stay healthy and protected.

Glutathione

This is a 3-amino-acid peptide (or tripeptide) consisting of glycine, glutamine, and cysteine. It is a vital antioxidant. When glutathione levels in cells drop too low, cell death occurs.

This is why glutathione is essential to the health of every cell in the body. It helps control inflammation, is critical for the immune system, boosts energy, and protects cells and tissues from free radicals—which protects you from disease. Furthermore, glutathione is important for optimal function of the five most important organs in the body: the heart, lungs, brain, liver, and kidneys. Glutathione is also required for optimal function of the immune system and for maintaining healthy eyes. Glutathione is considered the most abundant and most important antioxidant in the human body. One doctor calls it the "Michael Jordan of antioxidants and detoxifiers in the body."

What makes glutathione so effective and necessary? The secret of its power is the sulfur chemical groups (or sulfhydryl groups) in glutathione. Sulfur is a sticky, smelly molecule that acts like flypaper. Toxins stick to it and get trapped. In a body with a robust supply of glutathione, those toxins easily get trapped and then eliminated from the body. However, when glutathione levels in your body are low or become depleted, you can't effectively get rid of the toxins and can't effectively quench free-radical reactions. Thus you get a buildup of toxins and more damage to cells and tissues from free radicals, eventually resulting in disease.

Columbia University's School of Public Health stated that 95 percent of cancer is caused by a poor diet and excessive toxins.[2] Many patients with chronic disease have low glutathione levels. This long list includes fibromyalgia, chronic fatigue syndrome, autoimmune disease, heart disease, diabetes, cancer, Alzheimer's disease, Parkinson's disease, liver disease, kidney disease, and chronic viral infections such as HIV, AIDS, chronic hepatitis C, and chronic Epstein-Barr virus. Many patients with chronic disease also have a mutation of the glutathione gene, so they can't produce enough glutathione.

Phytosterols

One of the most important supplements in preventing colds, flu, and sinus infections is phytosterols. Sterols are plant fats that are similar to the animal fat cholesterol. All plants—including vegetables, fruits, nuts, and seeds—contain sterols and sterolins. These sterols play an important role in immune activity. Phytosterols can help T-cells multiply. In fact, one study showed T-cell response to this substance increasing from 20 percent to 920 percent after only four weeks on the sterol/sterolin mixture. Another experiment showed dramatic increases in natural killer cell activity. You can obtain phytosterols in an over-the-counter product called Moducare. Take one tablet three times a day, one hour before meals, or two in the morning and one in the evening on an empty stomach.

Beta-carotene

Beta-carotene should be taken once a day in a dose of 15 mg. Beta-carotene may come in dosages of 25,000 IU, which equals 15 mg (smokers should not take this supplement).

Chapter 10

KEEP MOVING

IF EXERCISE WERE a Hollywood star, she would fire her press agent for all the bad publicity she keeps getting. Yet the popular image of physical activity as some kind of grueling, forbidding obstacle course that will leave you gasping for air and sore for days is as outdated as the idea that you can get all the nutritional sources you need from modern food systems. For some people, just starting an exercise routine is incredibly difficult. However, once they start, they immediately begin to reap some of the benefits, which motivates them to continue. According to the US Public Health Service, physical fitness and exercise is one of the fifteen areas of greatest importance for improving the health of the public.[1]

Realize that you don't have to run marathons, spend hours in the gym, or lift backbreaking amounts of weight. Find a form of exercise that works well for you and stick with it. Bike riding, skating, jogging, dancing, or playing sports are just a few examples. For those who are elderly or have physical limitations, repeated forms of mild exercise—stretching or walking—can still help you tone up, feel good, and achieve a healthy body. When it comes to exercising in order to build your body's immune system, the watchword is: keep moving!

The first step in incorporating an exercise plan into your life is to make the commitment. It must be something that you have decided to do because you need to and something that you plan to stick with. Success requires time, effort, and patience. If you are a beginner, do not try to do too much too soon. Also, be prepared for it to take some time before you see the results. If you are willing to make the commitment and practice patience, you will see that it is far worth the reward.

Don't restrict yourself to a routine at home or in the gym either. Look for opportunities to move all day long. You can park farther from the store or other destination in order to give you a longer walk, take the stairs instead of the elevator, or toss a ball with your family in the backyard. Having fun is a key element to maintaining an exercise habit. Unless you prefer some solitude, try jogging or walking in the park with a friend. Think of recreational activities you can do with friends or family that don't cost much.

Powerful Benefits

Exercise will do more than boost your immune system. When you sweat a little, you are releasing stress, along with toxins that are stored in your system. The cleaner your body, the clearer your skin becomes. Combining exercise with plenty of fresh water and changing your diet to one that emphasizes more fruit and vegetables will make you look and feel better. And exercise is considered the best "nutrient" of all time. It can prolong fitness at any age and help you shed a few pounds too.

Exercise also helps increase your stamina and circulation, lifts depression, and increases joint mobility. Exercise actually nourishes joints. Bearing down or exercising a joint "stirs up" nutrients in the cartilage; movements cause the fluid to flow back into cartilage. This process can both nourish and lubricate the joints. Brisk walking, water aerobics, and stationary cycling are all good exercises for those who are dealing with arthritis or other causes of stiffness.

Then there is the impact on diabetes. As Dr. Reginald Cherry relates in his book *The Bible Cure*, in one study of twenty-two thousand people, those who exercised five or more times weekly had only 42 percent of the incidence of diabetes, compared to those who exercised less than once weekly. Those exercising two to four times a week had 38 percent of the incidence of diabetes, compared to those who exercised less than once weekly. Even those who exercised only once weekly had only 23 percent as high an incidence of diabetes as those who exercised less than once weekly.

Even folks who have conditions (such as arthritis) and fear that starting exercise will only increase their pain can follow a modified program. It could include deep breathing and stretching exercises in the morning to help limber up the body before getting outdoors for a mild walk. Taking a walk after dinner or walking on a treadmill will help increase blood circulation. Weight lifting doesn't have to be jerking a huge set of barbells in the air. Strengthen your arms and wrists by regularly curling a five-pound weight. Stretching before going to bed at night will help to relax you and promote more restful sleep. Work your way into this kind of regimen slowly. As you continue, you will see that you can walk faster and for longer periods of time with positive results. You will be surprised at how great it makes you feel.

A minimum of three times per week and a maximum of six times per week is a good schedule to follow; exercise for thirty to sixty minutes per session. Do the entire exercise at one time and keep your heart rate up, not allowing it to fall. One caution here: the nature of your body's health condition is complex and unique. Therefore, you should consult a health professional before you begin any new exercise, nutrition, or supplementation program, or if you have questions about your health.

Stimulating the System

One reason exercise is so helpful to strengthening your body is the ways it stimulates the circulatory and lymphatic system, raises metabolic efficiency, and enhances the body's natural cleansing ability. Conversely, a lack of exercise is a prime culprit in all kinds of problems. Poor circulation—which refers to sluggish blood flow through the body—can lead to such problems as heart attack and stroke. In addition to such factors as genetics, obesity, smoking, high blood pressure, and a high-stress environment, physical inactivity is one of the risk factors for coronary heart disease.

A lack of exercise can also contribute to the common problem of constipation. Many Americans have only three bowel movements a week. Now, the causes are varied and include such things as stress, a low-fiber diet, prescription drugs, or a poor diet with too much sugar, fast foods, and processed foods. But, technically, if you are not having a bowel movement at least once a day, then you are constipated and your bowels are sluggish. Bowel transit time should be twelve hours.

Exercise is vital for both protecting and maintaining a powerful immune system. Aerobic exercise—the kind that uses oxygen and increases your respiration and heart rate—is an excellent way to stimulate the immune system and help to prevent infections. Regular exercise will help keep your immune system strong and healthy. Regular aerobic exercise helps to decrease stress hormones and drain the sinuses by supplying more blood flow to the nasal area. It also increases mucous secretions so that stagnant mucus can be expelled from the sinus cavities.

Another way aerobic exercise works to keep you well is by raising your body's temperature. Heat actually activates the immune system. When you walk briskly or bike for about thirty minutes, your heightened temperature helps to stimulate the immune system. Exercise also oxygenates and strengthens tissues, making them more able to resist infection. As mentioned earlier, exercise helps eliminate toxins in the body. Your lymphatic system is vitally important in this elimination process, and it also helps to maintain your body's immune defenses. This system includes the lymph nodes, which are filters placed strategically throughout your body. Each person reading these words has about six hundred of them that systematically cleanse the body from disease. Lymph nodes contain white blood cells that scan the lymphatic fluid for bacteria, viruses, organic debris, and other microbes. These white blood cells contain much of the immune system's battalion of defense.

Macrophages, T-cells, B-cells, and lymphocytes attack enemy viruses, fungi, and bacteria.

When the lymphatic system becomes sluggish or blocked, the work of white blood cells slows down. This impedes their work of killing invading viruses, bacteria, and other microbes. As a result, infection and disease can more readily take root in the body. Nevertheless, regular aerobic exercise can supercharge this system, increasing its lymphatic flow threefold. That means three times as much cellular waste and foreign microbes are removed. This, in turn, greatly assists the immune system in its work.

Chapter 11

FOODS THAT HEAL AND
FEED YOUR COLD

I**N TODAY'S SOCIETY** it is becoming increasingly difficult to keep your immune system strong. The immune system is a complex system that depends on the interaction of many different cells, organs, and proteins for optimal function. Its task is to identify and eliminate foreign substances that invade the body and threaten our health. Vital components of the immune system include the thymus gland, bone marrow, lymphatic system, the liver, and the spleen.

A weak immune system leaves you more susceptible to illnesses, since it fights against many pathogens on a daily basis, such as yeast, parasites, fungi, and viruses. The immune system also combats antigens, such as pollen, chemicals, drugs, malignant cells, and more. The immune system is the greatest pharmacy in the world, making more than one hundred billion types of medicines known as antibodies to attack just about any unwanted germ or virus that enters the body. Best of all, the medicines made by this internal pharmacy do not produce side effects.

Your immune system has only one requirement: receiving the right raw materials to produce the internal medicines to safeguard you from illness. Frequent colds and flu are one of the indications that the immune system is not functioning at full capacity. Others include chronic respiratory problems, fatigue, allergies, yeast overgrowth, swollen glands, asthma, skin rashes, digestive complaints, and frequent headaches.

EATING FOR HEALTH

This is why eating healthy foods is a key to strong immune health. The legendary Greek physician (and father of modern medicine) Hippocrates practiced around 400 BC. He commonly used medicinal foods, such as apples, barley, and dates, to treat his patients. Hippocrates treated the patient and not the disease. Greek doctors Aristotle, Plato, Socrates,

Galen, and Paracelsus all used such methods as fasting, juices, soups, nutrition, and rest to bring their patients back to health. Hippocrates' saying, "Let your medicine be your food and let your food be your medicine," certainly applies.

For example, for years chicken soup has been called "Jewish penicillin." But now researchers are discovering what Jewish mothers knew all along: chicken soup can help a cold or flu. Hot chicken soup will actually help increase the flow of mucus and help clear out your sinuses. A 1978 study published in the journal *Chest* found that drinking hot chicken soup increased the nasal mucus velocity in fifteen healthy subjects from an average of 6.9 to 9.2 mm per minute. Chicken soup actually helps speed up the ciliary movement of the nose and bronchial passages so that they can eliminate microbes.[1]

Besides hot chicken soup, hot herbal teas, and vegetable broths, certain foods can also thin the mucus and stimulate its flow. Hot spicy foods, such as cayenne pepper, garlic, and horseradish, all help to clear nasal congestion and promote drainage. A Japanese horseradish called wasabi also promotes nasal drainage.

Quick Tips: The Power of Wasabi

Wasabi (wasabe), which is also called Japanese horseradish, comes from the root of an Asian plant. It's used to make a green-colored condiment that has a sharp, pungent, hot flavor and helps with nasal drainage from a cold. It can be found in specialty and Asian markets in both paste and powder form.[2]

With good eating habits, what you take into your body can promote your healing. As a brief reminder of earlier advice, you should eat as close to the "original garden" as possible, with plenty of fresh fruits and vegetables, high-fiber foods, seafood, yogurt, and kefir. Be sure to add garlic and onions to your recipes for added immune-boosting benefit.

You can overcome many infectious diseases by eliminating

mucus-forming foods, such as dairy products, eggs, and processed grains. The latter include pancakes, cereals, doughnuts, white bread, crackers, pretzels, bagels, white rice, and gravies. As advised in chapter 4, avoid sugary foods like cakes and pies, which depress immunity. Avoid fried foods, red meat, and refined foods as well. Also cut out of your diet margarine, butter, and other saturated, hydrogenated, and processed oils. Refined, polyunsaturated fats such as safflower oil, corn oil, soybean oil and so forth can impair immunity by interfering with the ability of white blood cells to fight infections.

Just as certain foods can help relieve the miserable symptoms of colds and sinus infections, other foods can work against you. Cold drinks, ice cream, and Popsicles can result in a buildup of mucus in the sinus cavities. In addition, eggs, chocolate, food additives, and excessive alcohol can trigger a buildup of mucus in many individuals. Setting up a guard nutritionally involves launching a campaign with two objectives: 1) building the wall, or strengthening your immune system with proper nutrition, and 2) eating foods that directly impact the symptoms of your cold, flu, or sinus infection.

The Mediterranean Diet

Recent years have seen a great interest developing in what is known as the Mediterranean diet. The diet followed by people living along the Mediterranean Sea results in some of the lowest rates of colon cancer, breast cancer, and coronary heart disease in the world. These kinds of results show how eating can literally heal you.

To examine some of the specific foods eaten by those in the ancient world can help you see how they help prevent and cure disease. It is no accident that Israel is one of these Mediterranean countries. Health experts believe that most of this diet can be traced back to the biblical guidelines given to God's chosen people—the Israelites. Mediterranean countries have developed their own dishes, but these dishes share several characteristics.

Quick Tips: Foods in Old Testament Times

When it comes to wise menu planning to fight colds and flu, take a tip from ancient cultures. Like many Arabs today, the Hebrews of thousands of years ago ate meat only on festive occasions. To vary the monotonous daily diet of parched or cooked wheat and barley, the Hebrew housewife would grind the grain into coarse flour, mix it with olive oil, and bake it into flat cakes of bread. She garnished the cakes with lentils, broad beans, and other vegetables. Cucumbers, onions, leeks, and garlic perked up bland dishes.

Fresh and dried fruit and wild honey sweetened the meals. In a water-short land the Hebrews heartily quaffed wine and prized the milk of goats and sheep. Solomon and his sumptuous court demanded richer fare for their golden table: "Solomon's provisions for one day was thirty kors of fine flour [about 335 bushels] and sixty kors of meal, ten fat oxen and twenty pasture-fed cattle, a hundred sheep in addition to deer, roebucks, gazelle, and fatted poultry" (1 Kings 4:22–23).

Take a glimpse into the everyday life of Mary, Joseph, and Jesus, and you will find that their dinner table held many of the same foods as those Solomon provided to his people: "In her daily rounds [the Jewish maiden Mary] she would have fetched water, tended the fire, and ground grain. The family dined on a porridge of wheat or barley groats, supplemented by beans, lentils, cucumbers, and other vegetables—with onions, leeks, garlic, and olive oil for seasoning. For dessert came dates, figs, and pomegranates. Watered wine was the universal drink. Only on feast days did humble Galileans eat meat."[3]

As you take a look at the ingredients used in these menus, you will observe that the following foods are consumed daily:

Olive oil. Olive oil replaces most fats, oils, butter, and margarine; it is used in salads as well as for cooking. Olive oil raises levels of the good cholesterol (HDL) and may strengthen immune system function. Extra-virgin olive oil is the preferred one to use.

Breads. Bread is consumed daily in dark, chewy, crusty loaves. The typical American sliced white bread and sliced wheat breads are not used in Mediterranean countries.

Pasta, rice, couscous, bulgur, potatoes. Pasta is often served with fresh vegetables and herbs sautéed in olive oil; occasionally it is served with small quantities of lean beef. Dark rice is preferred. Couscous and bulgur are other forms of wheat.

Grains. To obtain the same healthy grains, eat cereals containing wheat bran (one-half cup, four to five times weekly); alternate with a cereal such as Bran Buds (one-half cup) or those that contain oat bran (one-third cup).

Fruits. The Mediterranean diet includes many fruits, preferably raw. Eat two to three pieces daily.

Beans. This includes many kinds, including pintos, great northern, navy, and kidney beans. Bean and lentil soups are very popular (prepared with a small amount of olive oil). You should have at least one-half cup of beans, three to four times weekly.

Nuts. Almonds (ten per day) or walnuts (ten per day) rank at the top of the list of acceptable nuts in this diet.

Vegetables. Dark green vegetables are prominent, especially in salads. To obtain the same benefits in your diet, eat at least one of the following vegetables daily: cabbage, broccoli, cauliflower, turnip greens, or mustard greens; and one of the following groups of vegetables or fruits daily: carrots, spinach, sweet potatoes, cantaloupe, peaches, or apricots.

Cheese and yogurt. Unlike milk and milk products, some recent studies indicate that cheese may not contribute as much to clogged arteries as previously believed. In this diet, cheese may be grated on soups or a small wedge combined with a piece of fruit for dessert; use the reduced-fat varieties (fat-free kinds often taste like rubber). The best yogurt is fat free, but not frozen.

In addition to the healthy foods in the Mediterranean diet on a daily basis, there are some foods that you should include a few times a week. These include:

Fish. The healthiest fish are "cold-water" varieties such as cod, salmon, and mackerel; trout is also good. These fish are high in omega-3 fatty acids.

Poultry. Poultry can be eaten two to three times weekly; white breast meat from which the skin has been removed is the best.

Eggs. Eggs should be eaten in small amounts (two to three per week).

Red meat. Red meat should only be included in your diet on an average of three times a month. Use only lean cuts with the fat trimmed; it can also be used in small amounts as an additive to spice up soup or pasta. The severe restriction of red meat in the Mediterranean diet is a radical departure from the American diet, but it is a major contributor to the low rates of cancer and heart disease found in these countries.

Mediterranean Recipes

Here are several recipes that utilize many of the ingredients in this diet.

Recipe: Mediterranean-Style Bean Soup

1 Tbsp. extra-virgin olive oil
1 large chopped onion
3 medium peeled and chopped carrots
2 crushed garlic cloves
2 cups dried beans, soaked and drained
8 cups boiling water
1 14-oz. can stewed tomatoes with juice
1 Tbsp. fresh crumbled thyme (or 1 tsp. dried)
2 bay leaves
Approximately 1/4 cup chopped parsley, plus some for garnish
Morton Lite Salt and freshly ground black pepper to taste
Croutons for garnish (optional)

Soak the beans overnight, or prepare according to package directions. In a heavy three-quart stock pot, heat the olive oil and sauté the onion, carrots, and garlic until the vegetables are soft but not browned (about 10 minutes). Add the drained beans and boiling water to soup pot; add thyme, bay leaves, and parsley. Cover and cook over low heat 1 to 3 hours, adding water occasionally as needed or until beans are soft (cooking time varies with type of beans). When beans are soft, add the salt and pepper. For thicker soup, remove about 1 1/2 cups of beans and purée in a food processor or blender. Return to pot. For thinner soup, add hot water. Garnish with chopped parsley or croutons.

Recipe: Mediterranean Spinach Enchiladas

- 1 1/2 cups nonfat chicken broth
- 1 cup diced mild canned green chili peppers
- 2 diced tomatoes
- 2 Tbsp. finely chopped onions
- 2 cloves minced garlic
- 2 Tbsp. cornstarch
- 2 Tbsp. water
- 1 1/2 lb. fresh chopped spinach
- 8 corn tortillas

In a 2-quart saucepan, combine the broth, chili peppers, tomatoes, onions, and garlic. Bring to a boil. Simmer over low heat for 15 minutes.

In a small bowl, combine the cornstarch and water. Add to the broth and continue cooking, stirring as the mixture cooks until it thickens. Remove from the heat. While the sauce is cooking, steam the spinach for 5 minutes.

Coat a 9- by 13-inch baking dish with a no-cholesterol, no-stick cooking spray. Divide the spinach equally among the tortillas and roll, placing a single layer of enchiladas in the baking dish with the open side down. Top with the tomato mixture. Bake at 400 degrees for 10 minutes. This tasty dish will make a complete meal when served with a salad.

Recipe: Tabouli Salad

1 cup bulgur wheat

2 cups boiling water

3/4 cup fresh minced parsley

3/4 cup chopped green onions

3/4 cup cooked navy or garbanzo beans

1 cup diced cucumber

2 chopped tomatoes

3 Tbsp. fresh minced mint (or 1 tsp. each dried basil and oregano)

5 Tbsp. extra-virgin olive oil

5 Tbsp. fresh lemon juice

1/2 tsp. freshly ground black pepper

2 cloves minced garlic

1 small head romaine lettuce

Salad: In a glass or metal mixing bowl, pour the boiling water over the bulgur wheat. Cover the bowl and let it stand for 1 hour. Drain the excess water off the wheat. Add the parsley, onions, beans, cucumber, tomatoes, and mint. Set aside.

Dressing: Combine the olive oil, lemon juice, pepper, and garlic to make the dressing. Stir the dressing into the salad. Chill for at least one hour. Serve on a bed of whole lettuce leaves. Leaves may be rolled around the salad for eating as a finger food.

Recipe: Tomatoes Italiano

2 large halved tomatoes

3 Tbsp. shredded fresh basil (or 1 Tbsp. dried)

1-2 cloves minced garlic

Cracked black pepper

2 tsp. extra-virgin olive oil

Low-fat Parmesan cheese

In a small bowl, combine the basil, garlic, pepper, and olive oil. Spread equally on top of tomato halves. Sprinkle lightly with Parmesan cheese. Place in a round glass dish and microwave on high for 3 1/2 minutes. This is good with almost anything.

Recipe: Vinaigrette Dressing
_____

 2 Tbsp. red wine vinegar
 1/2 tsp. Morton Lite Salt
 1/2 tsp. dry mustard
 6 Tbsp. extra-virgin olive (or canola) oil
 1/2 tsp. freshly ground black pepper

Combine all ingredients. Whip dressing with a wire whisk until smooth. Pour over chilled lettuce, tomatoes, and other salad vegetables of your choice. Toss until well coated. Serve immediately.

Recipe: Garlic-Lemon Dressing
_____

 3 Tbsp. extra-virgin olive oil
 1 Tbsp. fresh lemon juice
 1/2 garlic clove
 1 tsp. Morton Lite Salt
 Freshly ground black pepper to taste

In a clean, dry salad bowl, crush the garlic and salt together with a spoon to make a smooth paste. Add the lemon juice and stir until the salt is dissolved. Add the olive oil and pepper. Mix the dressing well. This dressing, used in the eastern Mediterranean, is used on green salads as well as over steamed vegetables.

Chapter 12

DRINK YOUR WAY TO HEALTH

MANY AMERICANS SUFFER from aches and pains, constipation, skin eruptions, and fatigue. Such ailments put a strain on the body and its immune system. You may find it hard to believe that a simple lack of water is often behind these common health complaints. But our society consumes coffee by the gallon and soft drinks and iced tea by the liter. Plain old water for some people just seems boring or distasteful. Yet water is the original health beverage: no calories, no sodium, and no side effects. If you want to arm yourself in the battle against colds and flu, you can take a simple first step by substituting pure water for iced tea, coffee, concentrated juices, and soft drinks.

Your body cannot function properly without adequate water. Water makes up 65 to 75 percent of your body. It is second only to oxygen as an essential need for survival. Water helps to flush wastes and toxins, regulates body temperature, and acts as a shock absorber for joints, bones, and muscles. It cleanses the body and transports nutrients, proteins, vitamins, minerals, and sugars for assimilation. When you drink enough water, your body works at peak performance.

The recommended amount of water is six to eight 8-ounce glasses per day. If you have not been drinking water and this seems like a lot, start slowly and increase your intake gradually. Add a slice of fresh lemon, and you will get even more of a cleansing benefit. Water is easier to drink with a hint of flavor from a lemon. Plus, this combination can thin mucous secretions when you are ill.

SO MANY CHOICES

Once people catch a vision for the importance of water, their next question becomes what kind to drink. This is a valid concern; most tap water is chlorinated, fluoridated, or chemically treated to the point of being an irritant to the system instead of a blessing. Also, many toxic chemicals have found their way into ground water supplies. Growing concern about water purity has led to the huge bottled water industry. Many stores today have whole aisles dedicated to different kinds. Since this can create confusion, it may help to clarify the main options.

First, there is mineral water.

It most often comes from a natural spring with naturally occurring minerals. It has a taste that varies from one spring to the next. Naturally occurring minerals found in mineral water help aid digestion and bowel function.

There is distilled water.

You may have known someone who believes drinking distilled water is the only way to go. Some experts disagree. While distilled water is probably the purest water available, it is also demineralized. Drinking demineralized water on a long-term basis is not ideal, since your body needs the minerals that naturally occur in water.

There is sparkling water.

This choice comes from natural carbonation in underground springs. Most are artificially boosted in carbonation by CO_2 to maintain a longer fizz. Many people enjoy sparkling water after dinner as an aid to digestion.

If you choose not to purchase bottled water, you can purify your water by using a water filter in your home.

You can purchase water filters that attach to your kitchen sink faucet to remove impurities as water flows from the tap. You may also have noticed some water pitchers contain filters that purify the water as you fill them. Whatever type of water you choose, the most important thing to remember is that you must pay conscious attention to getting your quota of water every day. Thirst is not a reliable signal of a water need. You can easily lose a quart or more of water during activity before you feel thirsty.

Getting enough moisture into your body and sinuses is also a key factor in aiding your body to beat viruses. Water will keep your respiratory tract well hydrated and help liquefy any thick mucus that may be present during sinus infections. For sinus infections, colds, and flu, it is wise to increase water intake and drink at least two quarts (or more) of water daily. Also, get accustomed to drinking room temperature water instead of iced water or cold water. Cold liquids can actually impair normal respiratory function.

In addition to adequate water, keep enough moisture in your home; don't let it get dry during winter. Use a humidifier or keep a teapot simmering throughout the day to keep moisture in the air. For sinus pain, place a moist, hot cloth over your face.

Juice for Health

In addition to pure water, fresh juice will do wonders for your immune system. Why is reducing fresh fruits and raw vegetables to juice so beneficial for your body? Because drinking juices extracted from raw fruits and vegetables furnishes all the cells in the body with elements they need, and in a manner in which they can be easily and quickly assimilated. Fruit juices are the cleansers of our bodies, and vegetable juices are the builders and regenerators of our systems (think stronger immunity to colds and flu). Vegetable juices contain all the minerals, salts, amino acids, enzymes, and vitamins that the human body requires. This is why both fruit and vegetable juices are so important.

Another benefit of adding juices to your diet is that juices are digested and assimilated within ten to fifteen minutes of consumption. They are then utilized by the body to nourish and regenerate the cells, tissues, glands, and organs. The end result is positive because of the minimal effort needed by the digestive system to assimilate them.

One of the most important things to remember about juicing is to drink your juices fresh daily, when they are at their peak nutritionally. Plus, they spoil quickly. A caution: if you are ill or have a history of digestive difficulty, be sure to dilute your juice with water in a fifty-fifty mix. This will help prevent any bloating, gas, or other discomfort you could experience from ingesting this powerful liquid nutrition. Drink fruit juices at different times of the day than vegetable juices in order to prevent stomach upset. As a general rule, one pint daily is minimal for seeing positive results.

Essential Ingredients

In addition to water and easily absorbed protein and carbohydrates, freshly made fruit and vegetable juices provide a long list of essentials for your body. They include:

Protein

Since fruits and vegetables contain lower quantities of protein than animal foods, most consider them poor protein sources. But juices are concentrated forms of vegetables and fruit, and so provide easily absorbed amino acids. These are the building blocks that make up protein.

Carbohydrates

Vegetable juice contains carbs that provide fuel for the body, which it uses for movement, heat production, and chemical reactions. There are three categories of carbs: simple (sugars), complex (starches and fiber), and fiber. There are more simple sugars in fruit juice than vegetable juice, which is why you should juice more vegetables. Limit fruit juices to four ounces a day.

Essential fatty acids

There is very little fat in fruit and vegetable juices, but the fats juice contains are essential to health. The essential fatty acids (EFAs)—linoleic and alpha-linolenic acids in particular—found in fresh juice are components of nerve cells, cellular membranes, and hormone-like substances called prostaglandins.

Vitamins

Fresh juices are excellent sources of water-soluble vitamins like C, many of the B vitamins, and some fat-soluble vitamins.

Minerals

Fresh juice is loaded with these too. Minerals are components of enzymes that make up part of bone, teeth, and blood tissue, and help maintain normal cellular function. Minerals occur in inorganic forms in the soil; plants incorporate them into their tissues.

Enzymes

Fresh juices are chock-full of enzymes—those "living" molecules that work (with vitamins and minerals) to speed up reactions necessary for vital functions in the body. Without enzymes, we would not have life in our cells.

Phytochemicals

Plants contain substances that protect them from disease, injury, and pollution. These substances are known as phytochemicals—*phyto* means plant; *chemical* in this context means nutrient. Phytochemicals give plants their color, odor, and flavor. Unlike vitamins and enzymes, they are heat stable and can withstand cooking.

Biophotons

This substance, present in raw foods, is still being studied scientifically. Biophotons is light energy plants absorb from the sun and is found in the living cells of raw foods, such as fruits and vegetables.

Chapter 13

DETOX YOUR BODY

I F THE EARTH is sick and toxic, then there is a good chance it will impact your life. Unfortunately the toxic chemicals affecting people on a daily basis are difficult to see, smell, or taste. As a result, it is tough to avoid exposure to the thousands of toxins that slowly accumulate in your body. These poisons can eventually kill you through sickness and disease.

RELIEF THROUGH FASTING

One way to help your body get rid of toxins is to go on a fast. Periodic fasting can cleanse your body and both prevent and treat degenerative and other diseases. Fasting is a powerful, natural way to cleanse your body from the burden of excess toxins (such as toxic fats) and from many other chemicals and toxins. It is the best way to heal the body from degenerative diseases caused by overfeeding and poor nutrition. As Hippocrates, the father of modern medicine we quoted earlier, once said: "Everything in excess is opposed by nature." Not surprisingly, the United States is suffering an epidemic of degenerative diseases and death that is caused by excess. People have eaten too much sugar, fat, processed food, and empty calories.

Finding toxic relief through fasting can turn around your health and strengthen your immune system. Fasting gives your toxic, overtaxed body an opportunity to "catch up" with its overwhelming task of waste removal. Fasting allows your body to heal by giving it a rest—especially your digestive tract. Your body uses a significant amount of your energy every day in digesting, absorbing, and assimilating your food. When you give your digestive tract a chance to rest and repair, this also gives your overburdened liver a chance to catch up on its work of detoxification. All living things need to rest, including you.

Even the blood and the lymphatic system can be effectively cleansed of toxic buildup through fasting. During fasting, our cells, tissues, and organs can begin to dump out accumulated waste products of cellular metabolism, as well as chemicals and other toxins. This helps your cells to heal, repair, and gain strength. You have about sixty trillion to one hundred trillion cells in your body, and each one takes in nutrients and produces waste products. Fasting allows each cell to dump its waste products, allowing them to function at peak efficiency.

Fatty tissues release chemicals and toxins during fasting. These, in turn, are broken down by the liver and excreted by the kidneys. Your body will excrete toxins in many different ways during a fast (so be prepared if you experience some unpleasant side effects). Some people actually develop boils, rashes, or body odor during fasting since toxins are being released through the body's largest excretory organ, the skin.

Rejuvenate Physically

Fasting is also an energy booster. The toxic buildup in the cells and oxidative stress compromise the mitochondria so they cannot effectively produce energy. This leads to fatigue, irritability, and lethargy. This is because mitochondria are similar to tiny energy factories within each of your cells. Metabolic waste, chemicals, other toxins, and oxidative free radicals affect the function of the mitochondria of the cell, making them less efficient.

Periodic, short-term fasting will also strengthen your immune system and help you live longer. Deep cleansing of every cell in your body through fasting has the wonderful added benefit of improving your appearance. As your body detoxifies, your skin will eventually become clearer and glow with a radiance that you may not have seen for quite a few years. The whites of your eyes usually become clearer and whiter and may even sparkle. As toxic fat melts away through fasting, you will look and feel better than you have in years.

In addition, your mental functioning usually improves as your body cleanses, repairs, and rejuvenates itself. Given its powerful benefits, don't treat fasting as some horrible stretch of self-denial that relies solely on your willpower. Nor should you follow an unwise, "no food or water" routine, since total abstinence can be dangerous. Your body needs at least two quarts of water a day to sustain life.

Liver Friendly

Don't even try a water-only fast unless you are in good health, since this method can place considerable additional strain upon an already overworked liver. Since the liver is your primary detoxification organ, you need to do all that you can to support its vital functions. This is why a juice fast is preferable to a water fast. Freshly squeezed juices support your body's vital functions, while water fasting usually further depletes the liver of glutathione, a key detoxifier and antioxidant. That is one of the reasons for the overwhelming sense of fatigue you can experience during a water-only fast.

No matter what kind of fast you follow—such as juice only, or vegetables and fruit only—fast during a break or over a weekend, not when you are in the midst of a grueling work schedule. Also, talk to your doctor before initiating any kind of fast.

To prepare for a fast, you need to follow a liver-friendly set of preparations for two to four weeks. They start with avoiding cigarette smoke, alcohol, and drugs (set a goal of decreasing intake of all medications, although don't stop any prescriptions you need without consulting your doctor). If you take a lot of over-the-counter medicines, consider more natural ways to treat your various medical conditions, such as using vitamins and herbs. If you suffer from constipation, consider more natural ways to regulate your system, such as eating more fruits and vegetables, increasing fiber, or taking magnesium.

During this time you also need to avoid processed foods, refined foods, simple sugars (including honey), and fast foods (burgers, fries, pizza). Dramatically decrease your consumption of—or avoid—red meat, dairy products, and saturated fats like cheese and marbled meats. Eliminate trans fats; hydrogenated and partially hydrogenated fats (margarine, pastries, shortening); deep-fried foods; preserved and fatty meats; animal skins; processed vegetable oils; most salad dressings; coffee; colas; chocolate; and whipped toppings.

What can you eat? Choose organic fruits, organic vegetables, and free-range, organic, and lean or extra-lean meats. Eat as many raw organic vegetables as possible; when cooking vegetables, steam vegetables instead of boiling them. Prepared fresh organic vegetables are always better than frozen, and frozen are better than canned. Try preparing organic home-made vegetable soup too. However, avoid overcooking, and use as many fresh, raw vegetables as possible. Freshly juiced vegetables and fruits are great, as well. Drink a glass of freshly juiced fruits and vegetables in the morning instead of coffee.

Cruciferous vegetables, which we mentioned in chapter 5, are also essential. Certain vegetables are more important than others for liver detoxification. Ones you should eat often include cabbage, cauliflower, brussels sprouts, broccoli, kale, collard greens, mustard greens, turnips, and watercress. Other liver-friendly vegetables are legumes (all types of beans), beets, carrots, dandelion root, and dandelion greens.

Chapter 14

STRESS AND IMMUNITY

IN CHAPTER 11 we discussed how certain foods can help or hinder your immune system. In the same way certain foods can adversely affect the immune system, so can excessive stress. Stress is taking a toll on the American public's brain health and balance. Many people feel overworked, burned out, stressed out, and lacking desperately in "downtime." This isn't good. Stress depletes the brain and body of amino acids, the building blocks of protein, and of potassium. It hinders digestion, absorption of nutrients, and elimination.

While the causes and circumstances surrounding stress are very real, your reactions are equally important. Stress often involves your perceptions of events in your life more than the actual events. After all, one man can sit in his car in heavy traffic and whistle a tune while another one blows his stack. Stressful circumstances represent about 10 percent of a problem. Your reaction to those circumstances comprises the remaining 90 percent. Your perception and reaction to stressful circumstances will determine your immune system's response. If you respond to trying and difficult circumstances with faith, peace, and joy, your immune system will respond with strength. If you react by giving way to anxiety, grief, and fear, it will physically depress your immune system.

Quick Tips: Fighting Stress

Reducing stress is one way to strengthen your immune system. Here are some brief suggestions for lowering your stress levels:

- Simplify your life. Take inventory of how you spend your time, money, and energy, and determine whether you really want or need everything you currently invest in.
- Get enough sleep. Most people don't.

- Eat well.
- Exercise. It triggers chemical reactions in your body, enhances your mood, and makes you more capable of handling physical challenges.
- Have fun. Keep a good balance of work and play and of solitary and group activities. Sometimes you need time alone. Other times you need people around to hug, listen to, or share ideas.
- Maintain a support system. Make sure your schedule includes time with loved ones.
- Meditate and pray. Find ways to focus energy on a meaning and purpose beyond your everyday life.
- Be assertive. Don't bottle up negative emotions and experiences.
- Be creative. Indulge in enjoyable hobbies, such as painting, gardening, dancing, keeping a journal, or singing in a church choir (or by yourself).
- Give of yourself. Finding a way to help someone in need is the best way to remind yourself to be grateful for what you might take for granted.
- Pamper yourself. It doesn't cost much to relax with a long bubble bath, a foot bath while reading e-mail or mail, or with a series of family back rubs.

The latter can be especially hazardous to your health. If not addressed, chronic stress can take a serious toll on the body's immune system—whether it stems from marital strains, interpersonal conflicts, rebellious children, or strains in the workplace. Many can relate to this latter cause. Downsizing in industry and businesses stung by the recession—and in recent years reluctance to hire new employees—has prompted increasing numbers of employers to require more work from their employees, and with fewer resources. Not only have many employers pared benefits, but many also have reduced vacation time or other paid breaks. Then there is the effect of the electronic age, which keeps people tethered to work 24/7 via smartphones, Skype, computers, and other devices.

Whether personal, work-related, or a combination of both, these factors can create stress that causes your body to produce excessive amounts of cortisol. This in turn causes the thymus gland to shrink; this gland is vitally important for cell-mediated immunity and produces the critically important T-cells. Stress reduces the number of T-cells your immune system has to fight disease. It also decreases the numbers and the activity of natural killer cells.

In addition, too much cortisol in your bloodstream can impact the work of the lymph glands. The result of excessive stress chemicals in the body is that the immune system is no longer able to keep infections at bay. Stress opens the door for infections to enter into the body. This is like leaving your front door open all night and allowing any snake, possum, skunk, or rat to crawl in and set up a nest in your house. A similar thing happens with your immune system.

Adrenal Exhaustion

If stress has contributed to feelings of fatigue, it could be that your batteries need recharging. Pay attention to your adrenal glands. They are like two small batteries that sit on top of your kidneys and release hormones into your bloodstream. They are made up of two parts: the cortex, which is responsible for cortisone production, and the medulla, which secretes adrenaline. The cortex helps to maintain body balance, regulates sugar and carbohydrate metabolism, and produces certain sex hormones. The medulla's job is to produce epinephrine (otherwise known as adrenaline) and norepinephrine to speed up metabolism in order to cope with stress. When you are under stress, the adrenal glands increase your metabolism to ward off the negative effects.

Warning signs of adrenal exhaustion include severe reactions to odors or certain foods, recurring yeast infections, heart palpitations and panic attacks, dry skin and peeling nails, clammy hands and soles of feet, low energy and poor memory, chronic low back pain, and unreasonable cravings for salt and sugar.

One of the leading causes of problems with adrenal gland malfunctioning is too much stress. Among others are an A-type personality, consuming too much caffeine and sugar, vitamin deficiencies, or long-term corticosteroid use for asthma, arthritis, or allergies. Adrenal exhaustion is also common during the perimenopausal and menopausal stages of life. It is important to watch for warning signs of this debilitating condition. The main lifestyle change needed for improvement is plenty of rest, as well as moderated exercise like daily walking. Massage therapy also helps keep adrenals healthy by reliving stored stress and tension in the muscles and helping clear the adrenal pathways.

Adrenal supplements are available too. Pantothenic acid is a B vitamin known as an antistress vitamin that plays a role in the production of adrenal hormones; it helps alleviate anxiety and depression. A B-complex vitamin consists of the full spectrum of B vitamins, which help you maintain a healthy nervous system. Royal jelly, an antiaging superfood, is great for chronic fatigue and immune health. Astragalus (use as directed on bottle) is an herb that aids adrenal gland function, combats fatigue, and protects the immune system. You can also try Core Level Adrenal glandular supplement, which is available from a company called Nutri-West (use as directed by your health care professional).

MANAGING STRESS

There are many ways to deal with stress, starting with vigorous exercise. While you should consult your doctor about starting any exercise program, regular activity offers the benefits that more physically oriented generations gained automatically through physical labor. Exercise cancels out the effects of stress reactions on your body by draining off toxins. At the same time, you need to practice deep relaxation twenty minutes a day, since this helps neutralize the negative effects of stress.

Quick Tips: Stress Busters from Nature

If stress is weakening your immune system, try these natural stress relievers:

- Siberian ginseng: Siberian ginseng is a root that belongs to the ginseng family of adaptogenic herbs, which build resistance to stress. Siberian ginseng helps the body adapt to stress and lessens fatigue, often two underlying factors in anxiety.

- Valerian: Valerian is widely used in Europe as a sedative. It is said to be similar to benzodiazepine tranquilizers, but without side effects. Valerian works like benzodiazepines by enhancing the activity of GABA, the naturally tranquilizing neurotransmitter.

- Passionflower: Passionflower is a climbing plant, native to North America. Passionflower combined with valerian is a popular herbal remedy throughout much of Europe for insomnia, anxiety, and irritability.

- St. John's wort: St. John's wort has been used to treat anxiety and depression in Europe for more than twenty-four hundred years. It is a natural substance and enhances the activity of three important neurotransmitters: serotonin, norepinephrine, and dopamine. (Do not take St. John's wort if you are currently taking prescription antidepressants, especially MAO inhibitors such as Nardil or Parnate.)

- Kava: The root of Piper Methysticum, this member of the pepper tree is native to the South Pacific area. Kava has a natural tranquilizing effect on the brain by producing a soothing effect in the amygdala, the "alarm center" of the brain.

- 5-HTP: 5-HTP, derived from the seed of the Griffonia tree and related to the amino acid tryptophan, is used to treat anxiety, insomnia, depression, and other related conditions linked with low levels of serotonin.

Here are other suggestions to help you manage stress:

Recognize that attitudes and perceptions play a key role in managing stress.

Those dark scenarios you envision means you are probably over-reacting. Most things you fear never happen.

Maintain realistic expectations.

Many people manufacture stress by setting their expectations unrealistically high. This is especially true if you are a perfectionist. Plan bite-sized tasks you can do and check them off when finished, which will give you a sense of accomplishment.

Arrange your life so you feel in control.

You don't have to be in control of everything. You just need to feel you have some sense of control over your schedule and lifestyle. Plan how you will start to resolve dilemmas you face and tackle one immediately.

Build and maintain a support network.

This is the system that supports you in times of need and makes you aware that you are part of a bigger whole, toward which you have responsibilities. Support networks are particularly important when you are under stress.

Spend time with your loved ones.

Strong families tend to spend time together often. Unfortunately, when families get stressed out, a natural tendency is for the individuals to go off on their own or lash out against those close to them. Don't shoot down your allies!

Balance your commitment to your children, job, loved ones, and yourself.

Either too much or too little emphasis on self is unhealthy. Search constantly for that happy middle ground. Only you can determine the amount of stress that is healthy for you.

Other Methods

Massage

Massage aids in relaxation, gives relief from pain, and provides increased range of motion. Increasing demand for therapeutic massage is part of a trend toward health care with a mind, body, and spirit approach. Massage is one modality used to keep the body healthy, promoting relaxation and stress reduction. Massage therapy has become an integral part of health care and is frequently used by orthopedic doctors, chiropractors, and physical therapists. Massage helps to release physical and emotional tension.

Massage is the systematic and scientific manipulation of the soft tissues. Manipulations fall into four general categories: compressing, vibrating, percussing, and gliding. Massage physiologically relieves pain and metabolically prepares the injured or involved muscles for exercise or movement to their fullest capacity. According to research, massage does the following:

+ Improves blood circulation throughout the body

+ Helps relieve headaches

+ Helps break up adhesions and scar tissue

+ Aids digestive disorders, chronic fatigue, cardiovascular disorders, and gynecological problems

In addition, deep tissue and lymphatic drainage massage is a wonderful detoxification therapy, promoting elimination and drainage of mucus and fluid from the lungs.

Types of Massage

The popular types include:

* Swedish massage involves kneading, friction, tapping, and stroking to relax and cleanse the body. It helps muscles, nerves, joints, and the endocrine

system. It stimulates the body's circulation and will speed healing from injury.

- Alexander massage works to improve posture, expand the chest cavity, and improve breathing and body movement.
- Feldenkrais helps people to change the way they move and change unbalanced muscle patterns through body manipulation and exercise.
- Rolfing is deep manipulating of connective tissue.
- Polarity is based on the human body's magnetic field. The magnetic current and movement pattern is accessed to release blocks.

Hydrotherapy

Hydrotherapy is the practice of using hot or cold water therapeutically to improve many conditions, including stress, arthritis, headaches, menstrual problems, muscle pain, asthma, and back pain.

Osteopathy

Osteopathy is similar to chiropractic treatment, focusing on treating mechanical problems of the skeletal system. It is an effective treatment for many conditions, including stress, osteoarthritis, back pain, breathing problems, digestive problems, strain from sports injuries, and sciatica (back pain).

Quick Tips: Natural Stress Fighter

There are a number of methods for dealing with continuing stress. However, if you find yourself in an emergency stress situation, Rescue Remedy is a combination of wildflower essences formulated and recognized by Dr. Edward Bach, a medical doctor from Oxfordshire, England, who gave up his lucrative practice in the early 1900s to study the emotional links to ill health. He is recognized today as a pioneer in the field of mind-body medicine. In the 1930s Dr. Bach initiated a search for simpler, more natural medications than the vaccines he had previously formulated. He found them in the flowers growing around his pastoral college.

Rescue Remedy will help comfort, reassure, and calm you if you encounter troubling news, severe upsets, or startling experiences that can result in falling into a numbed, bemused state of mind. It can also be used just before bed to calm a troubled mind or before any stressful situation, such as exams, doctor or dentist appointments, or public speaking. Rescue Remedy also comes in cream form that can be used topically on burns, stings and sprains, or even as a massage cream.

Chapter 15

ESSENTIAL OILS AND AROMATHERAPY

I N THE LAST chapter we reviewed how stress can adversely affect the immune system and ways to address it. However, we reserved a separate chapter to review another way to combat stress: essential oils and aromatherapy. Stress reduction is an aromatherapy specialty, since this is a safe, pleasant way to lift your mood and relieve stress.

While aromatherapy may sound like a mystical, New Age–style treatment, it has proven scientific value. Smell is the most rapid of your five senses. The aroma of essential oil molecules works through hormonelike chemicals to produce healing results. Scents and odors influence the hypothalamus and other glands responsible for hormone levels, metabolism, and insulin. These glands monitor stress levels, appetite, body temperature, and even sex drive. When you smell an aroma, that sensual information is directly relayed to the hypothalamus (part of a large gland located near the center of the brain just below the thalamus and above the brain stem), where your motivations, moods, emotions, and creativity all begin. Different aromas evoke different responses as they influence your glandular functions.

Studies of brain waves show that scents like lavender increase alpha brain waves, which are associated with relaxation. Scents like jasmine boost beta waves, which are linked to alertness. Aromatherapy works by stimulating a release of neurotransmitters once an essential oil is inhaled. Neurotransmitters are brain chemicals responsible for pain reduction and pleasant feelings. This is a brief scientific explanation of how aromatherapy calms, sedates, and uplifts the body, mind, and spirit.

Ever wonder where the proverbs of our forefathers came from? Whether or not they understood the science of what they were saying, they knew it was wise to "smell the roses." Essential oils are most commonly used to counteract stress, which affects the mind and emotions. The effects of aromatherapy on the central nervous system are immediate and profound. In addition, aromatherapy gives a sense of well-being by releasing mood-inducing neurochemicals in the brain. Aromatherapy promotes relaxation, alertness, restful sleep, and physical relaxation. It can also increase energy. Aromatherapy has also been proven beneficial in helping prevent panic attacks.

Because the strength of essential oils is very concentrated, you should mix them with a "carrier oil" (such as almond oil) in a ratio of fifteen drops of aromatherapy essence to four ounces of the carrier oil. Just add a few drops of the essential oil and massage the body. You may also inhale them using a steam inhaler or a diffuser. Do not inhale them for more than fifteen minutes at a time. People with medical conditions, such as blood pressure problems or asthma, may have negative reactions to essential oils. Consult your health-care professional if you have any doubts about your condition.

Take a Bath

While taking a bath may sound like a routine matter, essential oils can turn this into an exercise in strengthening your body and immune system. If you want to make an attitude adjustment or uncover more energy, try a different aromatherapy bath each night of the week. You will be surprised at your fresher outlook on life. Some essences are stronger than others and are used for different effects, so count out just a few drops of some common scents and get revitalized.

Quick Tips: Body Work—Bathe to Relax

If you are suffering from too little sleep, high stress levels, poor diet, too much caffeine or alcohol, or frequent colds or flu, a therapeutic bath will alkalinize an over-acidic body. One therapeutic bath is a salt and soda bath, which counteracts the effects of radiation, whether from X-rays, cancer treatment, or other sources. Add one cup of baking soda and one to two cups of ordinary coarse salt, Epsom salts, or sea salt to a tub of warm water. (Keep bath to twenty minutes.) You will feel remarkably energized and refreshed. This should be taken periodically to keep your acid-alkaline level in balance. Pain and stress cause acidity in the body, which can translate into degenerative disease.

For maximum relaxation, enjoy a restful bath by adding to a tubful of water one of these essential oils: chamomile (two drops), cypress (five drops), orange blossom (two drops), or lavender (six drops).

If you are just beginning aromatherapy, try one or two of the following essential oils in your bath:

Restful bath

For maximum relaxation, add to a tubful of water one of these essential oils: chamomile (two drops), cypress (five drops), orange blossom (two drops), or lavender (six drops).

No-more-blahs bath

Try lemon (four drops), peppermint (four drops), basil (three drops), or bergamot (three drops).

Spicy bath

Feel fresh with geranium (three drops), lavender (six drops), juniper (five drops), or cardamom (four drops).

Wake-up bath

For a stimulating bath, use basil (three drops), peppermint (four drops), juniper (five drops), hyssop (three drops), or rosemary (five drops).

Tension bath

Ease your way through the end of the week with bergamot (three drops), geranium (three drops), or lavender (six drops).

A growing number of medical doctors believe that if more people used natural products like flower essences and aromatherapy oils, it would considerably lessen medical risks and side effects of more invasive or chemical (drug) therapies. It is a simple choice to make to see if your condition responds to these powerful natural therapies that many people find boost their health.

Choose Your Aromatherapy

Before we review some ways essential oils can help you fight colds and the flu, here are some oils that can help you deal with conditions that weaken your immune system and leave you susceptible to infectious diseases.

+ To deal with stress, lavender oil balances your nerves and emotions, calms the heart, and helps to lower blood pressure. Sandalwood is good for sleep and relaxation. Clary sage oil promotes feelings of well-being, calms your nerves, lifts the mood, and diminishes stress.

+ For depression, jasmine is an excellent natural method to address depression because it is uplifting and soothing. Lemon is also uplifting for the mood, while neroli oil relieves depression, insomnia, stress, and anxiety.

+ To boost your motivation and energy, ginger quickens and sharpens the senses and improves memory. Rosemary clears the brain and enhances memory. Peppermint is an energizer.

Cold and Flu Fighters

However, what about when you head into the cold and flu season? Essential oils can enhance the environment and keep your home free of germs. You can create an aroma lamp by filling a small bowl with water and five to eight drops of essential oil. Set it over a tea candle; the heat from the flame will evaporate the water, with tiny molecules of oil suspended in the water and filling the room.

As you inhale this mist, essential oils enter the nasal passages. This kills germs in the nasal cavity and bronchial tubes. These vapors also destroy germs in the air, such as those left by sneezing. You can use a variety of oils for this purpose, such as pine, rosemary, eucalyptus, camphor, cajuput, and lavender, which we listed above as an effective stress fighter as well. Another method for getting healthy oils into the air is to add some to a bottle of water and spray a mist into the room and around germ catchers like doorknobs.

You can also add oils to a humidifier to reduce germs as you freshen and moisturize the room. One reason you become more vulnerable to viruses in late fall and winter is that cool and dry air enables viruses to thrive. Low humidity dries out nasal passages and makes it harder for your body to trap and kill microbes. Some good tools for addressing colds are peppermint, which can ease headaches caused by congestion; oregano, an antibacterial agent that combats sinus infections; and eucalyptus, which is a decongestant and soothes respiratory problems.

Instead of reaching for a commercial mouthwash or other product, if you contract a sore throat you can use essential oils to make your own throat gargle (being careful not to swallow any of the solution). It only takes a drop or two of oil in a glass of warm water. Try eucalyptus, tea tree, garlic, or ginger for a great home remedy.

Oils—black pepper, hyssop, lemon, peppermint, or tea tree—can also address chills and a fever. You can put them on a cool compress and apply it to your head, or add a few drops to a bath.

Here are other ideas for using essential oils in the war with germs:

+ Dilute peppermint, lavender, or frankincense oil with a carrier oil and rub on the bottoms of your feet and spine.

+ Frankincense oil can be added to a homemade vapor rub and applied to the chest a few times a day.

+ To relieve congestion, mix two drops of pine oil, three drops of lemon oil, and three drops of eucalyptus with a carrier oil and sprinkle on a handkerchief or in a pint of water. Then breathe the vapors. Other oils that fight congestion are rosemary, peppermint, eucalyptus, lemon, lime, and frankincense.

+ Tea tree oil is a powerful antibacterial substance that can be mixed with water and applied to various surfaces to attack germs.

+ To stop a runny nose, place a drop of lemon oil on the side of your nose.

Chapter 16

GOOD HYGIENE

I N T H E F I G H T against colds and the flu, good hygiene is essential. The reason involves the ways viruses inflict infectious diseases on the human body. Once a virus gets transmitted to a person, it crawls inside to make contact with cells. The infection cycle begins when the virus attaches itself to cells. After attaching to the cell, these nasty invaders use the materials within the cell to duplicate themselves. They are released from the cell to go on to attach themselves to other nearby cells. Infection occurs as a result of newly formed viruses spreading to many cells.

Bacteria and fungi often infect specialized groups of cells in the body, called tissues. The skin, intestines, and kidneys are all examples of tissues that can get infected. The infection cycles of bacteria and fungi are quite different. They often travel through the bloodstream and associate themselves with the tissues. Once they have found their resting place, they begin to grow and multiply. Many bacteria can do this very quickly. Infection occurs as a result of many of these germs becoming associated with specific tissues. Parasites also attack specific tissues by locating in a place of residence and feeding off the tissue. They steal nutrients from the cells of the tissue they infect. Often, when they are cleared or released from the bodies of their host, they infect other individuals and start the infection cycle again.

Germs make you sick when your body tries to destroy the germs that infect it. The human body is an awesome creation whose immune system's sole purpose is protecting you from invasion and injury. The immune system recognizes when there is something present that does not belong. Like a combat situation, once it recognizes the enemy, your immune system does everything in its power to destroy or remove the enemy from your body.

GOOD HYGIENE PRACTICES

Realize that an ounce of prevention is worth a pound of cure. Simple, frequent hand washing is the most important thing that you can do to prevent colds, flu, and sinus infections. Indeed, this seemingly simple practice is the leading method of protecting against viral and bacterial infections. Why? Because you can catch—or spread—colds, flu, and sinus infections when you shake hands with someone, or when you touch an infected surface or object and then touch your nose, eyes, or mouth. Hand washing breaks this chain of infection.

In 2002 an article at CBSNews.com reported that over 100,000 deaths were linked to hospital infections in 2000. "Many of the deaths were caused by unsanitary facilities, germ-laden instruments and *unwashed hands*" (emphasis added).[1] The article mentioned an incident where a doctor dropped a surgical glove on a dirty floor, then picked it up and put it on his hand. He then changed the dressing on an open wound on a burn patient.[2]

Fast-forward to 2014, and CBS reported similar problems. The network cited a 2011 survey of 183 hospitals in ten states, published in the *New England Journal of Medicine*. That year there were 721,000 infections among 648,000 patients, with around 75,000 dying as a result of a health-care-associated infection. Again, CBS reported that many could easily have been prevented. It quoted Dr. Michael Bell, deputy director of the Centers for Disease Control and Prevention's division of health-care quality promotion, who said "patients can…take measures to protect themselves when they are in the hospital. This may mean verifying that your doctor has washed his hands, and even requesting the hospital run tests to ensure an antibiotic is actually working."[3]

Don't take a cavalier attitude toward washing your hands when using public restrooms either. They are a haven for microorganisms. After using a public restroom, it is important to wash your hands with hot water and soap. If available, use paper towels instead of automatic hand dryers. Do not touch the faucet when you turn it off; use the paper towel. Then, use the same towel to open the door or to turn the doorknob. Remember that all the previous visitors who didn't wash their hands on the way out have handled that doorknob.

While cell phones have nearly made pay phones extinct, some pay phones are still around many airports and bus stations. If you use one, you are holding the germs of everyone who has used that phone—right up against your mouth. It's best to handle public phones with a tissue or handkerchief, and keep the mouthpiece far from your mouth. Remember that they are breeding grounds for germs.

In addition, remember there is no such thing as an "innocent" handshake. It is an American custom to greet someone with a firm handshake. If we would bow as the Orientals do instead of shaking hands, it's possible that we wouldn't pass around nearly as many infectious diseases. During cold season it may be a good idea to carry antiseptic wipes with you and wipe your hands after shaking hands with individuals. Or make it a habit to wash them repeatedly throughout the day.

Cold viruses can typically survive for three hours on surfaces, on objects, and on hands. Viruses and bacteria live on our skin, and when we touch our mucous membranes, they easily gain entrance into our bodies. The simplest measure to prevent colds, flu, and sinus infections is to wash your hands frequently. The more often you wash your hands, the fewer colds, flu, and sinus infections you will get.

Showers and Saunas

Daily showering or baths are another essential in proper hygiene. Before you shower or bathe, consider brushing your skin. Because the skin is the largest organ in your body, brushing offers significant benefits. Use a loofah or vegetable brush, which you can purchase at a health food store. You need to brush all parts of the body away from the heart. Then follow this brushing with a sesame oil massage, which will bring a wonderful sense of relief. Massage the whole body for five minutes before bathing or showering. If you want to boost your healthful glutathione levels, take a cold shower daily or swim five to ten minutes a week in ice-cold water.

A very effective, inexpensive way to soothe sinus congestion and pressure is by simply replacing your showerhead with a shower massage. While taking a shower, set the shower massage on a pulsating setting and allow very warm water to pulsate over your sinus cavities. This provides dramatic relief for many sinus sufferers.

If you are a member of the YMCA or a health club, take advantage of the facility's steam bath. If you aren't contagious and don't represent a threat to others' health, steam baths are an excellent way to provide moisture to your mucous membranes and nasal cavities. However, if you can't go out, simply take a very hot, steamy shower and inhale the steam. It's very important to breathe the steam in through your nose to get the beneficial effects. You may also purchase a steam inhaler that uses a plastic mask that covers your nose and mouth.

If you have access to one, another fantastic way to cleanse your body is sessions in a sauna. Your skin naturally accumulates toxins and waste, even while showering in highly chlorinated city water. Sweating in a sauna produces amazing health benefits. It helps stimulate the release of accumulated toxins. This in turn increases your metabolism, reduces your appetite, promotes weight loss, and increases metabolic rate, which is the energy you expend while resting.

When you cleanse more frequently, impurities will come out of your skin. One of the best ways to speed up this process is to allow your skin to sweat out the toxins. Saunas are the best way to do this—especially the infrared kind. Any sauna will help, but infrared saunas go much deeper and offer a cellular level of cleansing. The deep heat penetration of infrared saunas removes not only toxins but also alcohol, nicotine, and metals. You burn more calories (up to 600 calories or more) sitting in this type of sauna for thirty minutes than you would running for a half hour. If you don't always have time to exercise, you can relax in a sauna and read a book or listen to music.

Infrared saunas also help with blood circulation, leaving you more beautiful, youthful, and with glowing skin. Many people have found pain relief for arthritis, back pain, muscle spasms, and headaches. Another benefit of infrared saunas is that they increase oxygenation and remove radioactive residues. They also are good for chronic infections.

Chapter 17

LIVE, LAUGH, LOVE

Y OU PROBABLY NEVER imagined that enjoying a good joke, watching a comedian, or taking time to frolic in the park with your children or grandchildren can help build your immune system and leave you less susceptible to colds and flu. Laughter, close familial relationships, and friends are part of the principles of healthful living that can strengthen your immune system. Social interaction and strong friendships keep emerging in research as important predictors of longer, happier, and healthier lives.

According to medical research, joy and laughter actually stimulate the immune system.

Loma Linda University Medical Center's Dr. Lee Berk reports that laughter helps the immune system in specific ways. For one, it increases IgA, which helps protect against respiratory infections, and gamma interferons, the immune system's frontline defense against viruses. It also increases B-cells, which produce antibodies directly against harmful bacteria. Laughter also boosts helper T-cells, which help organize the immune system's response. Finally, it raises the number and activity of natural killer cells, which attack tumor cells and viruses.[1]

Medical expert Dr. Don Colbert often prescribes ten belly laughs a day for his patients. Laughter stimulates the immune system better than most medicines and supplements and doesn't have any side effects. So, to strengthen your system, take Dr. Colbert's advice and build up your heart with laughter, joy, and frivolity. Life is too short to wear a frown all the time.

However, a well-rounded life includes more than enjoying some good laughs. While the image of rugged individualism has fueled countless movie heroes and the idea that "real men" (or women) go it alone, the truth is: life is tough. Everyone needs supportive coworkers, friends, family members, and a healthy balance of work and play. As we have reviewed in earlier chapters, you also need to make wise lifestyle choices.

Among them include stopping smoking, starting an exercise program, using massage therapy, getting early morning sunlight every day, and practicing deep breathing.

When it comes to emotional health, remember that those who fill their lives with laughter and maintain an optimistic outlook live longer and healthier lives. Not only is taking time to play and laugh important for long life, but also it will help defeat stress along the way. A sense of humor and hearty laughter release tension. Look for what's funny in everyday life. Find classic comedies on television, in the library's video section, or via Netflix or other on-demand video services.

A Well-Rounded Life

Here are some suggestions for achieving a rewarding life that will make you happier as well as healthier when cold and flu season arrives.

Build and maintain a working support network, which we mentioned in chapter 14 on stress.

This is the system that supports you in times of need and particularly in times of stress. One problem stress causes is tunnel vision, which is an inability to look at alternatives and options. Stress also makes you feel paranoid, as if people are out to "get you" or are purposely being difficult just to aggravate you. Share your perceptions with the important people in your life to see if you are seeing things clearly. Ask if they have any ideas about what you can do about it.

Spend time with your loved ones.

One of the healthiest things a family can do is to purposely spend some time together, go for a walk, or simply get out of the house and away from the TV or computer in order to do something fun outdoors.

Make time for your friends.

Time with friends can make life seem more pleasant, less stressful, and more fulfilling. A word here: if you constantly associate with people who put you down or constantly express cynical, critical, or negative views (and don't want to change), then find some new friends. Associating with positive people can propel you toward the successful person you want to become. "Guilt by association" is true. You will take on the positive or negative attributes of those you spend time with. When you hang around with angry people, you tend to be angrier than before.

Balance your commitment to your children, job, loved ones, and yourself.

Either too much or too little emphasis on self is unhealthy. Everyone needs to constantly search for that happy middle ground for self and family. In our previous discussion of stress, we pointed out that only you can determine the amount of stress that is healthy for you. One of the reasons stress can be such a killer is it often prevents you from having a good laugh and escaping life's daily pressures. Whatever is weighing you down isn't worth making yourself sick over.

Get adequate rest.

Even though we mentioned sleep in chapter 3, it is worth reminding you of the principle of getting adequate rest, which includes more than sleep. If you work nonstop seven days a week, you will burn out. You need to take a day to completely cut off contact with work, cell phones, computers, and other stress inducers. Originating with the Hebrew language, the word *Shabbat* means a once-a-week sabbatical. Seeing the benefits of sabbaticals have prompted some companies and other organizations to offer several weeks or even months off to long-term employees. While you may not have the opportunity for such an extended break, you can still spend one day a week resting, spending time outdoors, reading, or meditating as you listen to music. That day of rest will cause your other six days to be twice as productive.

A Positive Outlook

One reason for taking time to laugh is the way laughter can make problems and circumstances seem less daunting. A good belly laugh can counteract the negative impact of anger, rejection, fear, and bitterness, which all produce negative physical effects and release dangerous toxins into your body. Negative thoughts start to spiral you downward. You devote so much energy to these thoughts that you feel worn out and depleted. When you often dwell on negative thoughts, people can pick up on that and sense something negative. When your presence drains those around you, they tend to distance themselves from you.

If you live in a constant state of fear and anxiety, you are primarily hurting yourself by depleting your immune system. You will get sick much faster than those who don't live and think this way. Start to think on things that are helpful, exciting, positive, and energizing!

If you laugh and take a positive outlook on life, envision yourself achieving things, think the best of others, and dwell on positive thoughts, it helps rejuvenate your cells and improves your health. Your mind will send positive signals to your body.

Maintaining a positive outlook extends beyond yourself. People respond to external stimuli, so when others can visualize optimistic outcomes in present circumstances, it inspires them to push forward in their own lives. "Winners" are those who see possibilities, offer others hope, and help push people beyond their ordinary limits. They have overcome the innate human condition, which is to grumble, complain, and reason that things will never get better.

A Final Word

In chapter 11 we addressed the value of foods in strengthening your immune system. Besides choosing healthy foods, do your best to make mealtimes a joyous, pleasant social encounter. Celebrate family time by making menu planning, setting the table, and cooking together family activities. Make family and other meals about more than food too. Find purpose and fill your life with activities that are more meaningful than food. Volunteer at church, participate in an outreach program, call your family or your best friend, get involved with a passion or cause that you believe in—and dive in!

Chapter 18

GET OUTSIDE

WHEN IT COMES to building up your immune system, getting outdoors and enjoying a healthy amount of sunshine are two of your leading allies. Think of it as "nature's nurture." The sun is wonderful for your skin and is a vital source of vitamin D. The best time to get it is the morning sun, before noon. Sunshine activates your metabolism and speeds it up. These natural rays also diminish depression and reduce stress.

Thanks to our modern, climate-controlled, indoor environments with central heat and air, many people suffer from a sunlight deficiency. This is an unhealthy situation. Lack of exposure to sunlight slows your metabolism, leading to weight gain, possible depression, and increased appetite and overeating. Doctors recommend ten to twenty minutes a day of sun on your face and body.

Moderate sun exposure—with proper protection, depending on your skin type—will boost your immune system and ward off sickness and certain types of cancers. Safe amounts of natural sun exposure (ten to twenty minutes a day) will boost your vitamin D levels and improve your immune system. Spending time in the sun, coupled with a relaxing massage or a day at the beach, will relieve stress and change your outlook on life, strengthening you physically and mentally.

A key reason to get outside involves your body's physiology. Skin is the body's largest organ and is designed to eliminate toxins on a regular basis. A lack of sweating clogs your lymphatic system and slows metabolism. As much as you may love air-conditioning during a sweltering heat wave, you need to sweat to lose weight, shed toxins, and achieve good health. In reality, today's cooling systems are a modern-world-lifestyle deficiency. Coupled with a lack of regular sunlight, they are weakening your body.

Sick Building Syndrome

The need to get outside more often to get in touch with the sun and soil is seen through another modern-day deficiency related to office environments. Originally mentioned in chapter 1, it is known as "sick building syndrome." When a building's indoor pollution level rises this high, you are more likely to become ill with this illness, which is usually defined as "the occurrence of excessive work- or school-related illness among workers or students in buildings of recent construction." (The same can happen at home.)

If you work in a new office building you may think you are safer, but nothing could be further from the truth—new buildings are the worst. Volatile organic compounds, such as benzene, styrene, carbon tetrachloride, and other chemicals, are as much as one hundred times greater in new buildings, compared to the levels found outdoors. Building materials emit gasses into the air through a process known as "out-gassing." New carpets release formaldehyde. Paints release solvents such as toluene and formaldehyde. Furniture made from pressed wood releases formaldehyde into the air as well. In addition, such items as fabrics, couches, curtains, carpet padding, and glues are potential out-gassing sources.

The many chemicals released through out-gassing from carpets, paints, and glues can become so strong that those who work in these buildings can get seriously ill. With time, these toxic levels gradually decrease. Still, high amounts of volatile organic compounds are also around most offices. These compounds are emitted from copying machines, laser printers, computers, and other office equipment.

If you have been experiencing headaches that get more severe at work; experience itchy, red, watery eyes; experience a sore throat, dizziness, or nausea; or have problems concentrating, you may have symptoms of this syndrome. Among other symptoms are nasal congestion, shortness of breath, problems with memory and concentration, fatigue, and itching. While there may be nothing you can do about changing your work environment, you can make an effort to leave the building during lunch and on other breaks, and increase exposure to the outdoors when not at work.

Exercise and Walk

So, what should you do if you face such obstacles? A morning walk, run, or even a brisk swim for fifteen to twenty minutes before breakfast will help you start the day right. One reason is that when you wake up, your body is in a semi-fasted state and will burn fat right away. Then, later in the day, walk for thirty to sixty minutes outside. Involve your family in outdoors activity too. Go for a walk, ride bikes, play Frisbee at the park, or toss a ball around the backyard.

Whether as a family or individually, another outdoors activity you can do is barefoot walking. Walking barefoot in your garden or at a park will help you feel closer to nature and diminish stress. This will take your mind off everyday tensions, relax your body, rejuvenate your mind, and boost your energy levels. There are now special, minimalist-type shoes that have been designed to help launch your barefoot walking.

However you approach this effort, start slowly and gradually work your way up. At first, your feet will get sore quickly as the muscles are not used to being worked. With most shoes you walk with your heel first, but walking or running barefoot causes you to typically land on the ball of your foot toward the lateral side. Start by walking around the house barefoot or in your yard. Then try walking for maybe half a mile and gradually build up to longer lengths. It should cause an overall healing effect. It will connect you with the energy of the earth; diminish stress on your feet, legs, and body; and cause an overall feeling of relaxation and freedom.

In terms of an overall, individual exercise routine, you should strive to exercise at least three times a week with some type of cardiovascular workout—and if you can get outside to do it, so much the better. Even if you don't go for the barefoot variety, you will still feel more "grounded" when walking outdoors, since the earth is always moving and rotating. Walking outdoors keeps you in touch with the earth; indeed, the human body was made to walk. And when you get into the woods for a nature walk, you are much more likely to experience a sense of love, joy, energy, peace, and happiness than you would inside on a treadmill.

Even if weather doesn't permit you to head outdoors, exercise helps cleanse the body through sweating and improving blood circulation by elevating your heart rate. Exercise affects your hormones and body chemistry, which increases your overall sense of well-being.

GETTING AWAY

Keep in mind the benefits of nature the next time you plan a vacation. Whether camping, connecting with nature, swimming in the ocean, or going on nature hikes, you will notice that when you are on vacation in a natural setting, you feel more relaxed and under less stress. In this calmer environment you get fresh insights and inspiration. A major reason for this is the field of nature. Trees, rocks, and unspoiled forests carry a much higher energy frequency than metropolitan areas and downtown inner cities, where most everything is man-made and brimming with pollution.

Most artists enjoy natural surroundings in the mountains or on the beach, where they can seemingly tap in to a higher level of creativity. The closer you get to raw creation, the closer you draw to the Creator and the fresh, creative thoughts and abilities you would not otherwise experience. Most people living in stressful city environments consume less-than-nutritious, "dead" foods and swim in the shark-infested waters of urban life. Operating in survival mode, they fight traffic morning and evening in the ill-named rush hour, hoping to arrive home at a reasonable time—only to watch toxic TV or Internet programming that increases stress and cortisone levels.

For proof of what getting outdoors can do to improve your health, consider the residents of Okinawa, Japan. It is common for Okinawans to reach the age of 120 while still exercising, working, and enjoying life. Some health experts also credit their high intake of coral calcium from the ocean, as well as exercise and maintaining peace of mind. The latter stems from living more "connected" to the Creator's original designs for health, rest, and limiting the stresses and toxic lifestyles often found in major metropolitan areas. Part of the credit goes to Okinawans' healthy diets, which feature green and yellow vegetables and much less sugar and rice than other Japanese eat.

Chapter 19

KEEP YOUR NUMBERS DOWN

WHEN IT COMES to strengthening your immune system, you should never get too hung up on numbers. An unhealthy obsession over how many pounds you lost this week, how many miles you walked, how many calories you ate, or how many rock walls you climbed can prove self-defeating. Failing to meet predetermined goals can produce frustration, even depression, followed by resignation and throwing up your hands as you cry, "What's the use?" Then you stop trying to reach any health goals and sink into further danger.

While you should avoid falling into an obsessive/compulsive trap, at the same time you need to recognize that paying attention to key numbers is part of the battle against infectious viruses. The three you should keep an eye on are weight, cholesterol, and blood pressure.

Obesity and overweight conditions are familiar to most Americans, since they represent one of the United States' leading health problems. Data released in 2013 by the Centers for Disease Control and Prevention (CDC) showed that nearly 36 percent of adults ages twenty or older were obese, with a whopping 69 percent overweight. More than 18 percent of adolescents twelve to nineteen were obese; so were a similar percentage of children ages six to eleven.[1]

What's worse, childhood obesity in America has more than doubled in children and tripled among adolescents over the past three decades. The CDC says among the immediate health effects of obesity is the fact that youth are more likely to develop risk factors for cardiovascular disease, are more likely to have increased risk of diabetes in the future, and are at greater risk for bone and joint problems, sleep apnea, and social and psychological problems. Over the long term, they are more likely to be obese adults.

Too much weight can contribute to a host of other diseases, such as heart diseases, type 2 diabetes, stroke, and cancer. And it plays a major role in weakening your body and making you more likely to catch viruses. This is why we devoted chapter 11 to the topic of food and include many other references to eating throughout this guide. The CDC points out that healthy eating is associated with reduced risk for numerous diseases. One of the most important factors in achieving weight loss starts with the recognition of the link between losing weight and optimal health.

Quick Tips: Weight-Loss Tips

If you are concerned with shedding pounds as part of your goal of strengthening your immune system, here are some tips:

- Do not deprive yourself. An occasional slice of pie will not ruin your progress. Just remember, occasional is the key.

- Eat healthy (lots of vegetables, fruits, and whole grains daily).

- Ask for support. Make your friends and family aware of your weight-loss goal and enlist their help.

- Confide in friends and family, and God in prayer, to help work through personal problems so that you will not turn to food for comfort.

- Monitor your health. Heed any red flags such as constant fatigue, headache, and tension before they become full-fledged illness.

- Keep up with health screenings, blood pressure, cholesterol screenings, Pap smears, mammograms, dental checkups, skin exams, and chiropractic evaluations.

- Find purpose. Fill your life with things that mean more to you than food.

- Pray. A rich prayer life helps to decrease stress, low self-esteem, social pressures, and depression, all of which contribute to overeating.

- Get a diet buddy. If you're trying to change your daily habits without a little help from your friends, you might be missing a very important element.

Avoid Guilt

If you are struggling with your weight, don't get caught up in feelings of guilt, which will only compound the problem. Obesity is a complex and frustrating situation that has many causative factors. The list can include genetics, lack of exercise, overeating, stress, boredom, a low-fiber, high-carbohydrate diet, glandular and hormonal disorders, and age-related metabolic slowdown. If you ever heard senior citizens complain about the difficulties of losing weight, they aren't kidding—in advanced years, slimming down gets tougher.

While we have addressed healthy diets elsewhere, it is worth reminding you that a high-fiber diet is essential to good health. Fiber improves the excretion of fat, improves glucose tolerance, and gives you a feeling of fullness and satisfaction. This is why you should emphasize foods like brown rice, tuna, chicken, white fish, fresh fruits and vegetables, high-protein lean foods, lentils, and beans.

Remember to eat several small meals daily instead of skipping meals and eating one big meal daily. You want to give your body even-burning fuel throughout the day. If you "save up" for that gargantuan dinner, your body will store fat for "survival" instead of burning it. Remember to shun sugars and snack foods that contain salt and fat, such as potato chips, ice cream, candy, cookies, cake, sodas, and sugary breakfast cereals, as well as high-fat cheeses, sour cream, whole milk, butter, mayonnaise, fried foods, and rich salad dressings. And as we said in chapter 12, drink plenty of water.

The Lowdown on Cholesterol

High cholesterol can be defined as an excessive amount in the blood of the organic compound present in animal fats. It is also manufactured by the human body. Symptoms include cold hands and feet, difficulty breathing, heart palpitations, dizziness, high blood pressure, poor circulation, and fatigue. If you have experienced such symptoms, talk to your doctor.

Overconsumption of foods that are high in saturated fats and cholesterol, such as butter, eggs, cheese, heavy cream, and fatty meats, will raise cholesterol. Diuretics can also raise it by causing your body to excrete essential minerals. Mineral loss causes stress on the nervous system, leading to an increased need for adrenaline. Levels of cholesterol will rise in women who have difficulty converting cholesterol to estrogen and progesterone.

Just as wise eating habits can reduce weight, they can help cut cholesterol levels.

As with obesity and overweight problems, reducing high cholesterol means avoiding or limiting red meat, fried foods, full-fat dairy foods, and sugary and refined foods. The following will help lower cholesterol: garlic, high-fiber foods, fruits, vegetables, soy foods, olive oil, yogurt, and beans.

A Necessary Fat

Americans have been educated that they need to make sure their cholesterol levels are not too high because high cholesterol is considered a major factor in the development of heart disease. That is only part of the truth. Actually, cholesterol itself is not bad; it is a necessary fat made up of LDL, HDL, and several other components.

HDL is "good cholesterol" and keeps molecules from sticking to the sides of the arteries. LDL is "bad cholesterol," meaning it has sticky properties and can slow down the flow of blood to the heart, causing heart attack and death. Triglycerides are sugar-related blood fats that travel through the bloodstream along with HDL and LDL. High triglycerides also cause blood cells to stick together, increasing the risk of heart attack.

Previously we talked about how chronic stress can put a serious strain on your immune system. In addition, high levels of stress can cause an overproduction of adrenaline. Most hormones, including adrenaline, are manufactured from cholesterol. Therefore, when more adrenaline is needed, the body manufactures more cholesterol. Genetic predisposition (your heredity) can also cause high cholesterol. While you may not be able to change your ancestry, you can follow the other sensible steps just outlined.

What is a good cholesterol number? You should strive to keep total cholesterol under 160 mg/dl (and 130 is better), with your HDL in the 80–90 mg/dl range, and LDL in the 30–50 range. While 160–190 mg/dl falls in the high range, above 190 mg/dl is considered very high, and over 244 mg/dl means increased heart attack risk—not to mention related health problems.

BLOOD PRESSURE

Also known as hypertension, this condition is often called the "silent killer" because a person can suffer from high blood pressure and not have any noticeable symptoms. The exact cause is sometimes hard to pinpoint, as well. Contributing factors are heredity, high cholesterol, smoking, stress, high sodium intake, alcohol intake, and obesity. Secondary hypertension can be caused by pregnancy, birth control pills, diabetes, kidney disease, arteriosclerosis, congestive heart failure, and exposure to heavy metals. Symptoms include dizziness, headache, irritability, bloodshot eyes, and edema.

Your blood pressure is derived from a pair of readings. The "systolic" number is listed first and is the higher of the two. It is the measure of the pressure in the arteries when the heart beats and the heart muscle contracts. The diastolic is the lower, bottom number and measures the pressure in the arteries between heartbeats, when the muscle rests between beats and refills with blood. A reading above 140/90 indicates high blood pressure.

As with obesity and high cholesterol, eating can help you deal with this problem. You should eat a high-fiber diet, as well as adding garlic, celery, olive oil, and flaxseed oil to your menu. Avoid caffeine, since it raises blood pressure. Also, shun soy sauce, MSG, canned vegetables, smoked and aged cheeses and meats, chocolate, canned broths, and animal fats. Reduce your intake of salt; it promotes fluid retention, which increases blood pressure. Limit sugar intake as well, since it can increase sodium retention.

Lifestyle choices affect blood pressure too. You should use methods such as reducing stress, massage therapy, lavender aromatherapy, exercise, drinking hard water (soft water is high in sodium), and purchasing a blood pressure monitor. The latter can help you keep a daily journal of blood pressure readings to chart your progress.

While lots of people like to relax with a drink, remember that alcohol causes an immediate rise in blood pressure and adrenaline. Some of the supplements that can address high blood pressure are arjuna bark (500 mg three times daily); magnesium (400–800 mg daily); hawthorn (100–250 mg three times daily); vitamin E (100 IU daily); B-complex vitamins; calcium (1,000 mg daily); potassium (as directed on label); milk thistle for liver function; garlic (inhibits platelet aggregation); valerian root for stress; black cohosh, which calms the cardiovascular system; and cayenne, a blood pressure normalizer.

Chapter 20

WHEN TO GO TO THE DOCTOR

As you know, we are advocates of using natural methods to build up your immune system instead of automatically running to the pharmacy or taking antibiotics at the first sign of a cold or the flu. However, this doesn't mean you won't sometimes incur symptoms that require professional medical treatment. Allow wisdom and common sense to reign in your life instead of fear. For disease in general, risks can be greatly reduced by doing things that contribute to good health, including healthy eating habits and exercise. In addition, routine checkups by a doctor greatly increase the chances of successful treatment later for any kind of ailment.

When it comes to dealing with infectious diseases, sometimes going to your doctor or an emergency medical clinic is the best option. A word about doctors: they deal with treatments, which are remedies developed and prescribed to provide temporary relief for the symptoms associated with infection. A treatment differs from prevention in that it is designed to target the symptoms of a disease. Treatments do not prevent diseases from occurring. Physicians recommend treatments for illnesses, and often there are no guarantees. Doctors, after all, are human.

However, neither should you allow a cold or the flu to linger too long before you seek treatment. Tamiflu and Relenza are good prescription treatments for attacking the flu virus and preventing it from spreading. Also, treatment should begin within two days of the onset of symptoms. So don't foolishly try to "gut it out" if your fever has stayed at 101 or higher for a few days, you are unable to keep even chicken soup and crackers down, and your body is so weak you can barely get out of bed to use the bathroom.

Pay attention to your children's symptoms too. Some childhood illnesses seem unavoidable. Earaches and sore throats are great examples. If you have children or work with children, you have likely seen them

107

suffer from one, if not both, of these illnesses. For some children these infections occur frequently—so often, in fact, that their parents don't take them to see a doctor. However, even if a child gets these illnesses often, it is wise to see a professional. Earaches and sore throats are often signs of an infection. Infections always have the possibility of becoming complicated and causing severe illness if not treated properly.

Ear infections are especially common among young children. Infections of the throat affect most people by the time they reach adulthood, but some of the germs that cause these infections may also be carried on the skin and not cause symptoms. Both may also lead to severe complications if not treated properly. Sore throats are often symptoms of respiratory illnesses, such as colds, flu, and pneumonia, which is why you should not simply ignore them in hopes they will "go away."

Get Vaccinated

One way to keep trips to the doctor to a minimum is through vaccines, which can help prevent the spread of infectious diseases. Vaccines take advantage of your body's specific immunity. Once your body becomes infected with a germ, it can mount a specific immune response against it. While you may become ill the first time, with subsequent exposures to the same germ the body can respond more quickly because it "remembers" the germ. Usually, healthy people do not become ill when infected by the same germs at subsequent times in their lives. Essentially you become resistant, or immune, to those germs. This is the driving force behind vaccine development. A vaccine is a low or noninfectious dose of a germ that is given to provide protection by triggering a specific immune response.

Of particular note when it comes to cold and flu season is the flu vaccine. Although we noted earlier in this book that flu vaccines are not foolproof, that doesn't mean you should shun flu shots. The flu vaccine is an injection that contains killed viruses; therefore, you cannot get the flu from the vaccine. It actually contains three different strains of the flu virus. The strains that are chosen each year are the ones that scientists believe are most likely to be present in the United States that year.

If their choice is correct, the vaccine is 70–90 percent effective in preventing the flu in healthy patients under sixty-five years of age. The flu vaccine is recommended for adults and children over six months of age.

The flu vaccine contains the preservative thimerosal, which contains about 50 percent mercury by weight. There are thimerosal-free vaccines that your physician can order. Especially for young children, a thimerosal-free vaccine is a good idea. While many doctors also recommend the thimerosal-free flu vaccine for adults, adults are not nearly as susceptible to the harmful effects of thimerosal as young children.

It is recommended that you get the flu vaccine each year if:

+ You are a health-care worker.
+ You have diabetes, heart disease, or other long-term health problems.
+ You have a suppressed immune system.
+ You have problems with your kidneys.
+ You have a suppressed immune system.
+ You have a lung problem such as asthma or emphysema.
+ You are over fifty, and especially if you are over sixty-five.[1]

A second way to prevent infection with influenza viruses is to take antiviral drugs. There are a few antiviral drugs that are available for prevention of the flu; examples are amantadine and rimantadine. You should consult your physician before using this approach. Also, these drugs are prescribed early in the course of the infection, so you must see a physician immediately after symptoms appear.

Sinus Infections

A related infection that often accompanies a cold is a sinus infection. Colds and allergies (especially in children) are the most common triggers to sinus infections.

When you get a cold, your nasal mucous membrane becomes inflamed, swollen, and irritated. The entire lining of the nose and sinuses is covered with a thin coat of mucus. That mucus is sticky and collects airborne particles. It contains enzymes that destroy many bacteria.

The cilia are tiny hairs that line the sinuses and respiratory passages, which sweep away the debris that has been collected by the mucus out of the respiratory passages and sinuses. Anything that impairs the function of the cilia or the mucus can trigger a sinus infection. In addition, factors that cause the mucous glands to secrete more mucus or that create swollen tissues that block drainage can trigger a sinus infection too.

A cold virus shuts down the cilia, causing mucus in the nose to stagnate. Dry air from heaters and furnaces during cold winter months makes it worse. Cold air and frigid temperatures further irritate and injure the cilia, which is what triggers a runny nose. So you can see, many different factors work against the movement of the cilia and set you up for a sinus infection.

When mucous membranes become inflamed, swollen, and irritated, the mucous glands secrete even more mucus. Mucus normally drains easily through sinus openings, but if the membranes become swollen, irritated, and inflamed, the mucus can't drain out. It becomes stagnant and easily infected. If the mucus doesn't drain efficiently, the person will experience quite a bit of facial pressure, swelling, and pain over the sinus cavities.

Structural problems can also contribute to sinus infections. You may have a deviated nasal septum that hinders proper drainage. Nasal polyps inside the nasal cavity are growths that look similar to grapes and set up sinus infections by obstructing nasal drainage.

It's not clear why nasal polyps develop. Some may be caused by allergies, while others may be triggered by aspirin, chemicals, or even infections. But polyps commonly return. If you suffer from nasal polyps, your doctor may prescribe one of the new low-dose steroid nasal sprays, which are effective in keeping polyps from returning. Many factors can both cause and trigger sinus infections. By recognizing the irritating factors, you can then take measures to protect your cilia and mucous membranes from an assault.

Chapter 21

PRAY!

WHILE WE ARE leaving the topic of prayer to the last chapter, that doesn't mean it is the least significant method of strengthening your immune system. Because modern medicine was not available in biblical times, treating a sick person in that era involved making them as comfortable as possible and praying to God for healing. Today's medical advances mean doctors can do much more for patients than in days of old. Yet good doctors know the powerful role that faith and prayer still play in modern-day medical miracles. Even physicians who do not personally believe in prayer have to admit that people of faith often experience swifter healing and sustain longer-term recoveries than those without faith.

Indeed, prayer should be the first tool in your arsenal when infectious disease strikes. Most diseases have strong spiritual roots. Although traditional medicine often sees the body, mind, and spirit as separate, they are not. This is one reason prayer is a good method of preventing infectious diseases from even attacking you; for example, when it comes to recognizing signs of stress that can weaken your immune system, taking action early on to address the problem can include prayer, exercise, relaxation, and dietary changes.

MIRACLE HEALING

Prayer and healing are topics that provoke many myths and misunderstandings. The fact that God does heal some people instantaneously does not mean He does this every time. You should never limit God by placing expectations on Him of how He should, or will, heal you. Approach prayer with an open mind and heart. If you limit God by placing expectations on Him, you may completely miss what He wants to do in your situation.

The important thing is not to allow others who go to extremes sour you on the idea of miraculous healing. Dr. Richard Cherry, a renowned doctor in Houston, recalls how he learned about this soon after making a decision to follow Jesus. At the time, he was attending a small church that believed in God's healing power and praying for the sick. He observed people being supernaturally healed, including a woman with severe back problems. After people gathered around her, laid hands on her, and prayed, her pain suddenly disappeared. Dr. Cherry chalked it up to emotion that would quickly fade. Yet as the months rolled by and she remained healed, it confirmed God does indeed do this.

Later, at another church a man walked in one evening on crutches. No one laid hands on him or prayed for him, but the pastor said that God was healing someone with back pain and if he accepted that, he would be healed immediately. Then, as Dr. Cherry watched in amazement, the man on the crutches put them under his arms, ran down the aisle, and climbed up the steps to the platform. His family joined him and confirmed his disability, sharing how for years he had never been able to walk more than a few steps without excruciating pain.

"The man who had been crippled was now running all over the platform to demonstrate to everyone that God had really healed him," Dr. Cherry says. "I witnessed the awesome healing power of God. I agree with Jack Deere in *Surprised by the Power of the Spirit* when he contends that the real reason so many Christians do not believe in the healing power of God is 'simply because they have not seen miracles in their present experience.'[1] Before I witnessed these healings, I knew that Jesus healed in the Gospels, but I had not experienced His healing power today. But undeniable testimony of God's healing power happened right in front of me."

Pray and Ask

This experience helped Dr. Cherry formulate principles for finding healing, including praying and asking God for your healing. After all, if God can heal cancer, crippling conditions, and back problems, He is quite able to take care of cold and flu viruses.

One way to pray is to speak to the mountain obstructing your health. Pray specifically about the virus that has attacked you. Instead of praying, "God, heal my body," say, "God, I am praying that the infectious germs that have invaded my body be turned away. I know that You have created within my body an immune system with cells You designed and created to attack and destroy these viruses. Therefore, Father, I ask that You reactivate my immune system. In addition, Father, I ask that the Holy Spirit continue to guide me to truth as to everything I need to do in the natural to enhance and strengthen my immune system."

Once you have prayed this way, stand firm and have faith in God. If you check the tenth chapter of Daniel, you will see how this Old Testament prophet did just that. In Daniel's case he had to wait twenty-one days while God sent the archangel Michael to battle the forces of darkness to secure the answer Daniel's prayer. Now, a cold or flu that hung around for three weeks would be pretty serious stuff, but the principles you need to grasp hold of are patience and faith.

Also, realize that righteousness before God does not make you immune from attacks. The Bible says, "Many are the afflictions of the righteous, but the Lord delivers him out of them all" (Ps. 34:19). Yet you can rest assured that, even when you get attacked, God can help you overcome it. As John wrote, "You are of God, little children, and have overcome them, because He who is in you is greater than he who is in the world" (1 John 4:4).

Develop Prayer Life

Hearing, reading, and meditating on the Word of God and assembling with other believers in fellowship are all practices that will help develop your prayer life. In doing so, you will develop a closer relationship with God by learning about Him through His Word. You must become familiar with His will for your life, since it will enable you to pray and ask for His will to be done. You can pray for good health for yourself and loved ones in faith, believing—as Mark 11:24 says—you will receive what you ask.

Prayer is simply asking God to do what He promised in His Word.

For that to happen, you must become familiar with it. The only way to learn it and have faith in it is to hear it, read it, and meditate on it. Or, as Paul told the Romans: "So then faith comes by hearing, and hearing by the word of God" (Rom. 10:17).

Reading the Bible is a daily practice that every Christian should develop as well. There is no better way to become acquainted with the Word of God than to read it. While you may have struggled to understand the Bible in the past, there are many modern-language translations that make this easier today. Again, this is where a local church can help direct your study and understanding. A good pastor and church leaders can help guide you in the direction that you should go.

A Closing Prayer

If the discussion of prayer and spiritual life in this chapter has sounded foreign, but you would like to know Jesus, the Son of God and Savior of the world, we invite you to take this opportunity to meet Him. If you are ready to let Him come into your life and become your best friend, all you need to do is sincerely pray this prayer:

> Lord Jesus, I want to know You as my Savior and Lord. I believe You are the Son of God and that You died for my sins. I also believe You were raised from the dead and now sit at the right hand of the Father praying for me. I ask You to forgive me for my sins and change my heart so that I can be Your child and live with You eternally. Thank You for Your peace. Help me to walk with You so that I can begin to know You as my best friend and my Lord. Amen.

If you have prayed this prayer, you have just made the most important decision of your life. But don't keep this good news to yourself. Tell others what you have done, and find a Bible-believing church where the pastor and members can help guide you into this new and healthy phase of your life.

NOTES

Chapter 1—Know Your Environment

1. Jacqueline Krohn, *Natural Detoxification* (Vancouver, BC: Hartley & Marks Publishers Inc., 1996).
2. Centers for Disease Control and Prevention, "What to Expect From the Oil Spill and How to Protect Your Health," http://www.bt.cdc.gov/ gulfoilspill2010/what_to_expect.asp (accessed September 9, 2014).
3. Environmental Protection Agency, "Radiation Protection Basics," http://www .epa.gov/radiation/understand/protection_basics.html (accessed September 9, 2014).

Chapter 2—Know the Truth

1. S. Cohen et. al., "Psychological Stress and Susceptibility to the Common Cold," *New England Journal of Medicine* 325, no. 9 (August 1991): 606–612.

Chapter 3—Sleep and Rest

1. Robert Ivker, *Sinus Survival* (New York: Jeremy P. Tarcher/Putnam, 2000).
2. J. V. Ponike et al., "The Diagnosis and Incidence of Allergic Fungal Sinusitis," Mayo Clinic proceedings 74 (1999): 877–884.

Chapter 4—Limit Sugar Intake

1. Linda Page, *Healthy Healing*, 11th ed. (n.p.: Traditional Wisdom, Inc., 2000), 170.

Chapter 5—Superfoods That Build Immunity

1. K. A. Steinmetz et. al., "Vegetables, Fruit and Cancer. II. Mechanisms," *Cancer Causes & Control* 2 (1991): 427–442.
2. Paul Stamets, *Growing Gourmet and Medicinal Mushrooms* (n.p.: Ten Speed Publishing, 1994).
3. *Energy Times* (November/December 1999); *The Townsend Letter* (June 1998); Stamets, *Growing Gourmet and Medicinal Mushrooms*.
4. D. Ahn et al., "The Effects of Dietary Ellagic Acid on Rat Hepatic and Esophageal Mucosal Cytochrome P450 and Phase II Enzymes," *Carcinogenesis* 17 (1996): 821–828.

Chapter 6—Home Remedies for Colds and Flu Relief

1. Lynda Liu, "Fighting the Flu With Alternative Remedies," CNN, January 7, 2000, http://edition.cnn.com/2000/HEALTH/01/07/berrying.flu.wmd/index .html (accessed August 9, 2014).
2. Ibid.

3. Charlotte Mathis, "Chicken Soup, Ginger Tea, and Other Soothing Recipes for Colds," WebMD, http://www.webmd.com/cold-and-flu/cold-guide/chicken_soup_and_recipes_for_cold?page=2 (accessed August 9, 2014).

Chapter 7—Vitamins

1. Mavis Butcher, "Genetically Modified Food—GM Foods List and Information," Disabled-World.com, September 22, 2009, http://www.disabled-world.com/fitness/gm-foods.php (accessed August 9, 2014).

2. Linus Pauling, *Vitamin C and the Common Cold* (San Francisco: W. H. Freeman, 1970).

3. Linus Pauling, "The Significance of the Evidence of Ascorbic Acid and the Common Cold," *Proceedings of the National Academy of Sciences of the USA* 68 (November 1971): 2678–2681.

4. S. A. Glynn et al., "Folate and Cancer: A Review of the Literature," *New England Journal of Medicine* (1998): 1176–1178.

Chapter 8—Minerals

1. Sherif B. Mossad, et al., "Zinc Gluconate Lozenges for Treating the Common Cold," *Annals of Internal Medicine* 125 (July 15, 1996): 81–88; http://www.annals.org/cgi/content/abstract/125/2/81 (accessed August 9, 2014).

Chapter 9—Supplements

1. Page, *Healthy Healing*, A–317.

2. As reported in Sherrill Sellman, "The Total Body Cleanse Solution," *Total Health*, April 3, 2009, http://www.totalhealthmagazine.com/articles/body-skin-care/the-total-body-cleanse-solution.html (accessed October 31, 2014).

Chapter 10—Keep It Moving

1. US Department of Health and Human Services, Centers for Disease Control and Prevention, "Perspectives in Disease Prevention and Health Promotion Workshop on Epidemiologic and Public Health Aspects of Physical Activity and Exercise," *Morbidity and Mortality Weekly Report* 34, no. 13 (April 5, 1985): 173–176, 181–182; http://www.cdc.gov/mmwr/preview/mmwrhtml/00000513.htm (accessed August 9, 2014).

Chapter 11—Foods That Heal and Feed Your Cold

1. K. Saketkhoo et al., "Effects of Drinking Hot Water, Cold Water, and Chicken Soup on Nasal Mucus Velocity and Nasal Airflow Resistance," *Chest* 74 (October 1978): 408–410; http://www.ncbi.nlm.nih.gov/entrez/query.fcgi?cmd=Retrieve&db=PubMed&list_uids=359266&dopt=Abstract (accessed August 9, 2014).

2. Sharon Tyler Herbst and Ron Herbst, *The Food Lover's Companion*, 4th edition (Hauppauge, NY: Barron's Educational Series Inc., 2007), s.v. "wasabi."

3. J. Pritchard, ed. *Everyday Life in Bible Times* (n.p: National Geographic Society, 1967), 242, 332.

Chapter 16—Good Hygiene

1. Brian Dakss, "Hospital Infection Deaths in Focus," CBSNews.com, July 21, 2002, http://www.cbsnews.com/stories/2002/07/20/health/main515755 .shtml (accessed August 9, 2014).
2. Ibid.
3. Jessica Firger, "In U.S., Hospital-Acquired Infections Run Rampant," CBSNews.com, March 26, 2014, http://www.cbsnews.com/news/in-us -hospital-acquired-infections-run-rampant/ (accessed July 14, 2014).

Chapter 17—Live, Laugh, Love

1. Lee Berk, "Eustress of Mirthful Laughter Modifies Natural Killer Cell Activity," *Clinical Research* 37 (1989): 115.

Chapter 19—Keep Your Numbers Down

1. Centers for Disease Control and Prevention, "Obesity and Overweight," http://www.cdc.gov/nchs/fastats/obesity-overweight.htm (accessed August 9, 2014).

Chapter 20—When to Go to the Doctor

1. Influenza Vaccine, FamilyDoctor.org, http://familydoctor.org/x2084.xml (accessed December 30, 2003).

Chapter 21—Pray!

1. Jack Deere, *Surprised by the Power of the Spirit* (Grand Rapids, MI: Zondervan Publishing House, 1993), 57.

BIBLIOGRAPHY

Content from this book was adapted from the following previously published Siloam books:

Calbom, Cherie. *The Juice Lady's Big Book of Juices and Green Smoothies*. Lake Mary, FL: Siloam, 2013.

Cherry, Reginald. *The Bible Cure*. Lake Mary, FL: Siloam, 1998.

Colbert, Don. *The Bible Cure for Colds and Flu*. Lake Mary, FL: Siloam, 2004.

———. *Toxic Relief*. Lake Mary, FL: Siloam, 2012.

Dauphin, Leslie Ann. *The Germ Handbook*. Lake Mary, FL: Siloam, 2005.

Maccaro, Janet. *Natural Health Remedies*. Lake Mary, FL: Siloam, 2003.

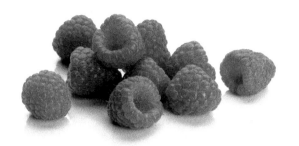
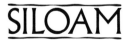

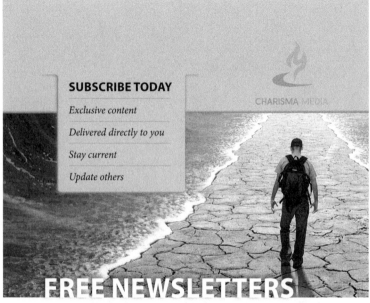